the LOW CARB MYTH

Free Yourself From Carb Myths, and Discover the Secret Keys That Really Determine Your Health and Fat Loss Destiny

By: Ari Whitten

www.ariwhitten.com

&

Wade Smith, MD

www.qangl.com

Publishing services provided by Archangel Ink

ISBN: 1942761643
ISBN-13: 978-1-942761-64-8

Table of Contents

Foreward

Many years ago, I asked a wise, older friend of mine why he talked so much about food with other people. He told me, "Everyone likes to eat, and talking about what you like to eat makes people happy. Instead of talking about topics that everyone argues about, I stick to food, which keeps the conversations friendly."

My how things have changed! In this day and age, discussions about what we should eat and why are as controversial as politics and religion. There are so many opinions with many individuals quoting scientific studies and many touting their own self-study, which is usually based on suffering through deprivation diets and poor food choices. The state of discussion regarding food, health, and diet has escalated to a frantic level of opinion, bias, and name-calling that can only mean one thing: there is a lot of money in getting people to follow a specific diet philosophy!

Consider also that in the million or so years of hominid and human evolution, we are currently in the first epoch of time when humans need to read books in order to figure out how to eat and live a reasonable life. Why is this so? The reasons are varied and include the availability of information via the internet, a media-promulgated obsession with physical appearance, and the current concept that all of us can live to be 105 without disease if we just do everything right.

On the other hand, the plethora of diet research and health information—easily available to consumers—is enabling global changes in eating habits and improved lifestyles that hopefully will manifest in lowered rates of obesity, chronic disease, and disability.

The problem is that so much of what is quoted as science is often misquoted and misunderstood, or is not really good science. As a physician, scientist, scientific editor, and writer, I can share with you that the insider view of science is that you have to read each study carefully and somewhat objectively, because most of what gets published is not very definitive. What you cannot and should not do is read and believe only that which supports your thesis or opinion. Many of the current philosophies regarding diet and health use scientific data to justify conclusions that are simply incorrect once you read the data carefully. In many cases, the data is not all wrong, but the conclusions of whichever diet guru's book you are reading are overblown. This phenomenon in medical editing and publishing is known as making strong conclusions that are supported by weak data. A relevant example in the diet world is the concept of low-carbohydrate diets being genetically suited to humans due to the "fact" (actually not a fact, in any manner) that humans prior to about 10,000 BC ate very little starch. This particular assumption has tremendous, romantic, "noble savage" imagery, especially in the chaos of modern Western cultures. The corollary to the Paleo assumption is that prior to human agriculture and grain eating, humans mostly looked like Olympic decathlon athletes and lived long satisfying lives without the torture of chronic disease. Since no hunter-gatherers in today's world look like Olympians or live longer than other groups, the main data to support these suppositions is the fact that human genomes have not changed more than one percent in 15,000 years. Therefore, whatever we were 15,000 years ago must be what we should be now! This type of fact manipulation serves the mythological need of humans to look at the distant past as a source of mystical truth, but drawing conclusions with such little data and such few facts is NOT science.

I have spent many years as a competitive athlete, coach, physician, and researcher observing the effects of diet and health practices on human performance and, most importantly, on human health. As an orthopedic trauma surgeon, I have been particularly concerned with rehabilitating patients after severe injury and helping them to find balance in their lives. The ongoing influence of diet books, diet trends, and various "experts" is unmistakable and not entirely positive. Based on research and experience treating patients, I began offering the advice to "eat as if you owned an organic farm next to an ocean. Eat what you could grow, catch, or kill, but most importantly, eat what you like and what makes you feel well." However, more often than not, the patients or athletes we were counseling were trying to carb load and eat low fat in the 70s and 80s; and in the 90s, 2000s, and on, they are experimenting with low carb or Paleo. Neither of these approaches stands up to the test of time or to scientific analysis. The low-carb approach is the most insidious and dangerous, however, due to the complexity of science surrounding human hormones and the ease with which the public can be impressed with out-of-context scientific quotes.

We should note that recent studies on low-carb diets have shown that they are effective in short-term weight loss and do not increase the risk of cardiovascular disease in the short term, despite high levels of saturated fat. The weight-loss effects are no different from those of non-low-carb diets with equal calories. In other words, low-carb diets help people lose weight primarily because they limit calorie intake, the same way low-fat or other diets do. Additionally, some low-carb diets such as Paleo encourage increased vegetable intake and elimination of refined carbohydrates and processed food, which may be a huge improvement in nutrition compared to standard Western diets. Low-carb diets, in some cases, are a stepping-stone towards healthier and more balanced eating. However, low-carb diets are not magical fat-burning diets that turn on our genes to replicate the robust, perfect health of humans unpolluted by modern living! They are also not long-term diets for those with significant energy requirements such as laborers, children, pregnant women, athletes, those with high-stress jobs, or those with reasonable activity levels. Of all the patients and colleagues I have observed on low-carb diets, the only ones who could stay relatively low carb were those with sedentary lives. And most of these "supplemented" with high-carb alcohol and "cheat days." Most people are overstressed, micronutrient deprived, under- or over-exercising for their lifestyle, suffering from irregular sleep, and trying to make up for it all by eating a special diet. The special diet of the times is low-carb, which makes little sense historically or scientifically but makes a lot of sense in terms of book sales, websites, and seminars. After years of extreme diet recommendations for unpalatable low-fat food, is it any surprise that we all say "Yay!" when we are told the secret to our lives is to eat bacon and rib eyes?!

Thankfully, despite the ubiquity of low-carb diets, there are sane voices that have observed through long-term experience that low-carb diets are not sustainable for most people, that the science behind them is contrived and misinterpreted, that no documented, long-lived cultures eat low-carb, and, most importantly, that common sense and the successful history of humankind tells us that we are not necessarily genetically programmed to restrict a specific macronutrient.

Ari Whitten is one of these sane voices. His rational approach to diet, exercise, and health is based on *scientifically sound* genetic and evolutionary principles. We have teamed up to help those suffering from imbalanced diets caused by the current focus on weight loss and low-carbohydrate eating. While we recognize that the human race can eat just about anything and keep reproducing and growing and that with seven billion people on Earth, some are going to feel great eating mostly meat and fat and some just as great eating mostly starch, the great truth for most of us is in the middle. We look forward to giving you the facts, good and bad, about eating. The preponderance of evidence, experience, and common sense points to carbohydrate eating in humans as being perfectly congruent with good health and body composition. For those struggling with the opposite viewpoint, we offer you *The Low-Carb Myth*.

Wade Smith, MD

How to Read This Book

Before you start reading this book, it's important to be aware that this book presents a great deal of scientific information. For many readers who are less interested in nutritional science and physiology than in the nuts and bolts of healthy eating, there may be sections of this book that some might find too dry, too "sciency," or simply overwhelming.

We have spent countless hours condensing, synthesizing, and *simplifying* all of this science so it is accessible and understandable to the lay reader—that is, *as easily understandable as possible.*

This book is, in fact, not intended as a textbook for nutrition experts. Rather, it is intended for the general reader interested in health and nutrition. However, the science underlying all of the myths that have been perpetuated about carbohydrates and insulin is *complex*. This complexity is a reality, whether we like or not, and while most things can be explained in straightforward language, there are still many aspects of the science that require detailed analysis of the scientific literature.

We have done our best to follow the idiom, "Things should be made as simple as possible, but not simpler."

That is, we have striven to distill complex topics into understandable concepts and language without distorting the scientific and physiological reality, which is frequently complex.

Moreover, there are really two audiences that this book must speak to:

1) Low-carb advocates who will no doubt read this book wanting to argue with everything, looking for holes in the logic and science in order to go on supporting their preconceived dogmas. (Many followers of low-carb dogma will go to great lengths to attack anyone who suggests that carbohydrates are not the scourge of the world and that low-carb diets may not be as beneficial as they wish to believe. So we fully expect such people to read this book solely for the purpose of looking for any reason to write a negative review and defend the honor of their chosen diet.)
2) The general reader, who, with best intentions, adopted a low-carb diet and has since failed to experience the health and fat-loss benefits that were promised by those promoting that low-carb diet. Perhaps this reader is also experiencing *negative* effects and simply wants to learn why and to find their way out of the mess.

Speaking to the second group, which is of much greater importance, requires straightforward facts and explanations.

Depending on who you are, your current level of knowledge of the science around these topics, and your level of interest in that science, you will likely want to read this book in very different ways.

If you're not interested in all the scientific details, please don't feel as though you have to read through every word of every section. Instead, skip around to the specific sections that interest you. The scientific nature of this book—referencing over 400 studies—combined with the fact that readers will have diverse interests and levels of knowledge regarding the science of nutrition and physiology makes it such that not all readers will find all sections to be easy reading or particularly enjoyable. **Please do not force yourself to read through sections that you find uninteresting! The bottom line is that this is *not* a novel, and <u>you *do not* have to read through this book in sequence from beginning to end</u>.**

Each chapter stands on its own, and thus, you can feel free to skim through this book to the specific sections that you're interested in learning about. While the chapters do build on one another to some extent, each chapter is designed to stand largely on its own and can be read separately.

To summarize:

- If you're a reader well versed in the scientific literature, feel free to read every page of each section, and read the studies for yourself. If you want to feast on the scientific details and controversy, feel free to do so!
- If you're a lay reader without a science background, but you are interested in understanding the science, read every page of each section.
- If you're a lay reader without a science background, you have little to no interest in getting wrapped up in all of the scientific minutiae, and you are interested in just the actionable conclusions, please read the beginning of each chapter and then skip to the chapter summaries at the end of each chapter to learn the take-home message in a very time-efficient and easy-to-understand way.

With a book such as this one that presents a huge amount of dense scientific material, it's easy to get bogged down in the scientific minutiae and never arrive at the sections that are ultimately of interest to you. So, **if you're interested in just the practical, take-home messages and don't want to get bogged down in all the details of the science, we recommend that you do <u>not</u> try to read the book from cover to cover.** To make your reading experience enjoyable, we strongly suggest that you skip over sections where the information is less interesting to you, skip directly to the summary sections as desired, and, in general, use the table of contents to skip around to the specific chapters and specific topics that *do* interest you. **For those not interested in all the scientific details, this will be the difference between finding this book very boring or completely fascinating.**

It's all in *how* you read this book.

Introduction: Everything is "Scientifically Proven" to be Bad for You!

There are hundreds of thousands of studies that have been conducted on innumerable aspects of human nutrition. The sheer volume of information and data is astounding. Perhaps even more astounding is the simple fact that no matter what one's personal beliefs about nutrition, it is possible to support one's nutritional philosophies with scientific studies to "prove" that that approach is superior.

If you are so inclined, you can find studies to help you demonize diets rich in protein. You can find studies that help you demonize high fat intakes. And you can find studies that help you demonize carbohydrates.

If you want to get more nuanced, you can also find studies that allow you to paint a picture that *certain kinds* of proteins, fats, and carbohydrates are uniquely bad. You can find studies that imply that saturated fats are bad, or polyunsaturated fats, or perhaps specific kinds of polyunsaturated fats. You can find studies to say that animal proteins are harmful while, say, soy protein isn't, or that animal proteins are safe while soy is harmful. And you can find studies that imply that fructose is bad or sucrose is bad or starch is bad or high-glycemic carbohydrates are bad.

It is possible to find dozens of studies to support any of those innumerable different stances, and as long as you cherry-pick the studies and ignore all the ones that conflict with your position, you can give the appearance that your stance is unassailable "*scientific truth.*"

This sort of pseudoscience is rampant and takes many forms:

- You have vegans who think eating a diet of nothing but green vegetable juices, salads, grains, legumes, nuts, and seeds is optimal for health (your average vegan); other vegans who think humans are meant to eat nothing but fruit (Dr. Doug Graham of "80/10/10 Diet" fame); and people like Dr. McDougall (of *The Starch Solution* diet fame) who think humans should eat basically nothing but starch foods. All are convinced that animal foods are the devil.
- You have low-fat advocates who think any fat they consume will give them diabetes or heart disease and make them obese.
- You have the low-carb dieters who think any carbs they eat "turn into fat" and otherwise make them sick and diseased, not to mention their belief that eating carbs will turn them into "sugar burners" and prevent them from accessing the "preferred" metabolic state of being a "fat burner."

But the most amazing part of all this is that no matter which one of these schools of thought you subscribe to, you can find very convincing scientific evidence to support your belief system.

Let us show you how preposterous the conclusions can be, based on the vast amount of contradictory health and diet information that exists in the published literature and on the internet.

Oh my god, I feel like I've really stumbled on to some amazing information. I've been eating carbs and sugar all these years, but now I have discovered why I haven't been that healthy lately and why I've been putting on more weight over the last few years. Dr. Mercola says that sugar is a poison that wrecks your health and is even more addictive than cocaine! I just found out from this UCLA study that "sugar lowers your IQ and shrinks your brain." And don't even get me started on fructose! Don't you know fructose is toxic to your liver just like alcohol? At least, that's what Dr. Robert Lustig's video on YouTube told me. This documentary called Fed Up, *along with Gary Taubes' book,* Good Calories, Bad Calories, *told me that sugar is the cause of all our obesity and diabetes woes. See, the low-carb Paleo people are right! Carbs really are the devil!*

Wait, hold on just one minute. It appears that actually FAT is the real toxic macronutrient. Look, I can find hundreds of studies that show that fat damages your brain and causes diabetes and obesity! Here are just a couple examples: High-fat diet injures the brain. High-fat diets cause insulin resistance and diabetes. High-fat diets cause Alzheimer's. High-fat diets cause obesity!

And that is just a tiny fraction of the studies I found. Countless other studies in rats and humans have shown that high-fat diets induce obesity and all sorts of nasty diseases. So maybe it's fat that is the real devil here.

Hmm, so at this point, it appears that both fat and carbs are toxic to the human body...

So I guess we should only eat protein, since that is the only thing left—you know, if we can't eat either carbs or fat.

But, oh no, I just got some bad news. It turns out that if you eat too much protein, it will shrink your brain and cause Alzheimer's! And according to T. Colin Campbell's The China Study, *it will even give you cancer!*

Yikes! I guess no fat, no carbs, and no protein is the way to go.

Let's see... What does that leave us? I guess we should just eat nothing but green vegetables, since that's pretty much the only thing left.

Perfect. I guess I'll just eat green vegetables, since that's mostly just fiber and vitamins and minerals.

Oh, except many green leafy vegetables are high in oxalates, which can damage your organs and glands if you eat too many of them. And cruciferous vegetables, if eaten raw, are goitrogens—that is, they screw up your thyroid function.[1] [2]

So, I'm not really sure if we can have any of this stuff at this point—carbs, fats, proteins, and even green vegetables all seem bad for us.

Maybe we should just drink water? That is pretty much the only thing left...

BUT, water seems to be even more toxic than fats, carbs, or protein!!!

How many deaths are there from people eating too many carbs or fat or protein? None. But how many are there from overconsuming water? LOTS! It turns out that drinking too much water at once is extremely bad for you. It can cause irreversible brain damage and can even kill you! (Seriously. Click the links to see the studies if you don't believe me!)

So better not drink any water, either!

Oh, and don't even get me started on the sun!

I just found out that the sun emits harmful UV rays that can damage your skin and give you cancer!

Better avoid the sun, too!

So, if you want health, my recommendation based on the science is no carbs, no fat, no protein, no veggies, no water, and no sun for you!

---

1 http://www.ncbi.nlm.nih.gov/pubmed/8819891

2 http://www.westonaprice.org/basics/bearers-of-the-cross#goitrogens

The purpose of this seemingly silly exercise is to illustrate a simple but very important point: any of the essential nutrients of life can be villainized—even with the appearance of being "scientifically proven" to be harmful—if one is so inclined to cherry-pick and misrepresent the data to serve that purpose.

This little exercise is also meant to illustrate that there is a fine line between a medicine and a poison. You can take *any* required nutrient for human health (even *water*) and find "science" to say that it's "bad for you."

Unfortunately, this sort of cherry-picking is far too common in the world today—even among health gurus.

This brings us to a very important point that is absolutely critical to understand and take with you as you read the rest of this book: **there is a hierarchy of scientific evidence.**

What does that mean?

It means that there are different levels of evidence that distinguish claims that have poor scientific support from claims with the highest levels of scientific support. You simply *must* understand this if you are going to effectively navigate the crazy, mixed-up world of health gurus giving all sorts of conflicting advice. There's just no way around it.

To ground all of this in something practical, consider what category you might lump the following two claims in—poorly supported claims vs. strongly supported claims:

1) "Everything happens for a reason."
2) "The earth is round."

The first statement may perhaps be true, but there is zero objective scientific data to support the statement. The second statement is a known fact validated by the highest levels of concrete scientific observation and data. For someone to say that these are two equally proven facts (or equally *unproven*) would be utterly ridiculous.

Unfortunately, in the realm of nutrition, the distinctions are not so clear cut. Most of the claims of the superiority of one type of diet or another lie between the two extremes—there may be some fragment of truth in the claim, but usually the claim is far from the whole picture. Because of the strong biases that various health authors have about their way of eating, we are often told that their way is scientifically proven, even though, just like "everything happens for a reason," the facts do not support the claim.

This may seem like an unimportant point, but it's absolutely critical to grasp this hierarchy of evidence—particularly in a field like nutrition—in order to effectively distinguish poorly supported claims from solid scientific evidence.

In short, this is the blueprint for knowing whether or not someone is cherry-picking the data.

With that said, let's take a very brief look at how this hierarchy actually works.

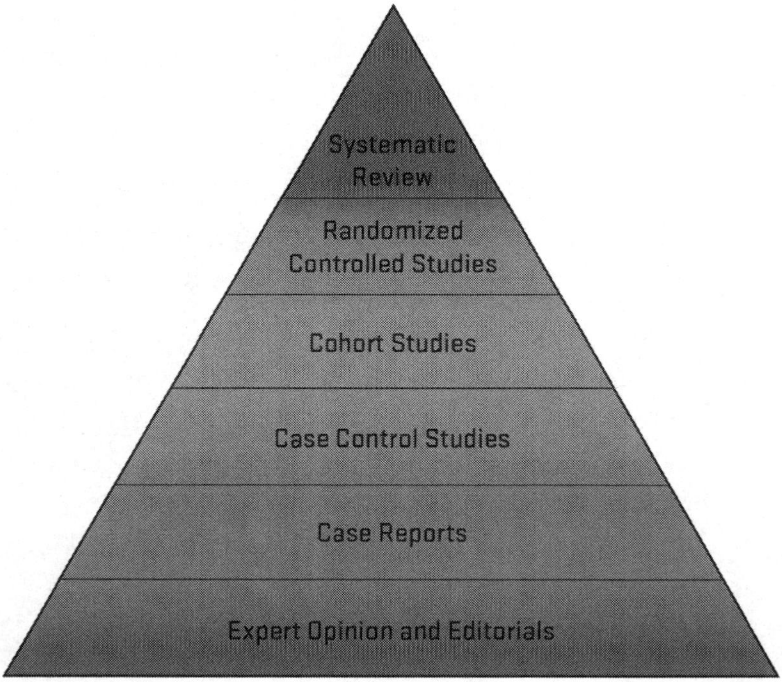
Systematic
Review
Randomized
Controlled Studies
Cohort Studies
Case Control Studies
Case Reports
Expert Opinion and Editorials

The lowest level of evidence that is considered meaningful is the opinions of scientists and experts in a given field. Above that is case reports, then case-control studies, then cohort studies (observational series), and then significantly above that are randomized controlled trials (RCTs). At the top of the hierarchy of evidence—the strongest level of evidence—is systematic reviews.

When it comes to nutrition, we need to think of the hierarchy of evidence like this:

- **One study—no matter how well designed and well controlled—proves almost nothing!** Even three single studies prove virtually nothing. Yet, we frequently see otherwise intelligent people taking one study and using it either to "prove" their own preconceived dogmas or "prove wrong" others' dogmas. Why is this such a problem? Consider this: If all it took was one or two studies to "prove" something, it would quite literally be possible to go back through the annals of research and establish the most ridiculous versions of reality imaginable by citing at least one study in support of it. Now, one study can absolutely be pointing to the truth in a matter. One well-done, well-designed study can make a big point, send researchers in the right direction, and potentially change the way we look at things. However, for that study to be a bona fide game changer, it must be repeated, verified, and retested by independent professional scientists (and it must also *not* have numerous other studies that contradict it). This is the standard for any major scientific finding, whether in the fields of medicine, engineering, social sciences, or nutrition. In the field of nutrition in particular, one study—or even a handful of studies—is not nearly enough to make any sort of broad conclusion.
- **Well-supported claims are the realm of the *comprehensive literature review*. A comprehensive literature review on any subject is a compendium of *all* of the studies conducted on that particular subject--"all" being a critical component in order to prevent cherry-picking.**
- Beyond even that, when multiple lines of converging evidence (from numerous comprehensive literature reviews) from multiple related scientific fields all point to a particular set of conclusions, we can establish something as near-incontrovertible scientific evidence (i.e., as good as scientific evidence gets). The extreme example of this would be "the earth is round." Countless lines of evidence support that

> conclusion, while—and this is important—little to no evidence contradicts it. That's the level of evidence that we want to be striving for.

The main point to keep in mind is that virtually all of the individual studies that have compared so-called "low-carb diets" to other types of diets like "low-fat diets"—even the most well-controlled and long-term studies—are actually not significant evidence (in and of themselves) of *anything*. These are but a tiny sliver of the pie.

Nutrition is a complex science with a slippery mess of confounding variables lurking under the surface of almost everything we want to test. Even in the best-controlled nutrition studies, there are almost always one or two confounding variables that cause people to draw incorrect conclusions if they try to make broad statements from that study. Exactly what these confounding variables are will be explained in detail over the course of this book, but for now, **the important thing to understand is that in the field of nutrition, to have real evidence of something and to prevent cherry-picking of the data, we need to be operating at the level of systematic reviews done on large bodies of well-controlled RCTs, not engaged in silly battles with each group adhering to a particular type of dietary dogma while cherry-picking their handful of studies to "prove" their approach is the best.**

In this book, we argue that the science of nutrition is so complex that we need to consider not just systematic reviews comparing low-carb to low-fat diets, we need to integrate larger bodies of evidence from nutritional science to generate logical explanations that account for *all* of the data.

This is a critical point. One study isn't enough—even a randomized control study. Even a handful of RCTs or comprehensive literature reviews aren't enough either. We need to examine all the dozens of systematic reviews from multiple related fields, go into the hundreds of RCTs, and look at numerous lines of epidemiological evidence—assess every angle of the data—to generate something meaningful enough to draw strong conclusions. We need comprehensive explanations that can account for *all* of the data—not more selective presentation of the evidence to support one's pet theory, while ignoring the mountain of evidence that contradicts it.

That is precisely what is *not* being done by most health and nutrition gurus out there. The health and fat loss industry is chock full of people who are all too willing to forgo any understanding of the hierarchy of evidence and selectively pluck a handful of studies to "prove" their theory is correct, while ignoring large bodies of contradictory evidence and comprehensive literature reviews that conflict with their beliefs.

Where does this lead?

It leads directly to the situation we're in now: countless health "gurus" out there all preaching radically different diets—most of which are extreme, unsustainable, promote ideas that are in contradiction to large bodies of evidence, and frequently cause harm to the health of those who follow them—while quoting a few studies to give the impression that their approach is the one true "scientifically proven" approach.

This cacophony of conflicting recommendations is mirrored by the incredible confusion among the general public, who are told that grains are good, then that they are bad; that vegetable oils are good, then they will kill you; that soy is good, then it is bad; milk is good, milk is bad; fat is the main dietary devil one decade, and carbs the next… ad nauseam, ad infinitum.

This is truly a mess.

To find our way out of this mess requires combing through thousands of studies and examining all of the most relevant systematic literature reviews, countless RCTs, the consensus opinions of renowned obesity and nutrition scientists, and myriad lines of epidemiological evidence, and then taking each tiny sliver of the pie, putting the pieces together, and making sense of the enormous body of evidence that results.

We propose that the confusion and seemingly "contradictory" information out there in the realm of nutrition is not so much the result of truly contradictory scientific evidence. To the contrary, the evidence is actually far clearer than most imagine. Rather, the confusion is mostly the result of deeply flawed interpretations and cherry-picking of the evidence by people who put "proving" their own theories ahead of challenging their own preconceived dogmas through objective and thorough analysis of the data.

To be clear, however, reading and interpreting scientific data is not easy. Performing scientific research is a full-time job that is difficult and requires years of rigorous training. Even many people who are excellent at jobs that require scientific education, such as doctors, engineers, and pharmacists, have deficits in their ability to critically analyze and interpret the scientific literature. The reason is that their job generally does not require regular analysis of research, and they usually have not undergone specific training to learn those skills. This does not mean that *only* research MDs and PhDs can critically analyze and interpret scientific literature. But it does mean that we should be careful in accepting the advice of health gurus with minimal formal scientific training, who claim that their personal reading of scientific research has revealed some wonderful truth that everyone else has missed, which is at odds with the mainstream opinions of scientists in that field. At best this is delusional, and at worst, misleading others for money.

This sort of pseudoscience—lack of understanding of the hierarchy of evidence, ignoring large bodies of contradictory evidence, and seeing only what one wishes to see—is, to a large degree, precisely the sort of "science" that the low-carb movement has been built upon.

The concept that humans are designed by evolution to eat minimal-carbohydrate diets and that such a diet leads to the pinnacle of health is a misconception built on a foundation of inaccuracy, half-truths, cherry-picking, and misrepresentations of the scientific data.

These carbohydrate myths and half-truths are not harmless. We have seen countless people infected with this low-carb pseudoscience who are now afraid to eat fruit or potatoes because they think the carbohydrates contained in those foods will "turn to fat" or that they'll end up with diabetes, obesity, or some other severe health problem. Despite an overwhelming amount of data to the contrary, many have been persuaded that these low-carb mythologies are true.

In the same way that low-carb gurus have demonized carbohydrates through selective presentation of the scientific data, we can do the exact same thing to give the impression that the high-fat, high-protein diets they advocate are infinitely worse than the high-carbohydrate diets they attack. This is not at all difficult to do. In fact, there are literally *thousands* of studies that implicate high-fat diets as causing everything from heart disease to brain damage, to inflammation, to depression, to diabetes, to Alzheimer's, to obesity. For every study that one uses to try to say that sugar promotes fat gain or diabetes or damages the brain, we can find two studies claiming the exact same thing about the effects of a high-fat diet.

However, the point of this book is not to replace one myopic war on a single macronutrient (carbs) with a new myopic war on a single macronutrient (fat).

Nor is the point of this book to convince you that low-carb diets are universally harmful. In fact, there are some circumstances where a low-carb diet is potentially appropriate. Nor is the point of this book to say state that no one has ever improved their health or lost fat by following a low-carb diet—indeed many people *have* profoundly improved their health and body composition on low-carb diets. (So if you or someone you know has gone on a low-carb diet and improved their health and lost a large amount of body fat, rest assured that we are not denying that such effects do occur. Yet, it is important to note from the outset that while some low-carb diets may provide certain benefits, many of the fat loss and health benefits people attain are *not* actually due to the reasons that many low-carb gurus claim! Rather, it is for other hidden reasons—which will be explained in detail later in this book—that don't have to do with the inherent metabolic effects of carbohydrates or insulin.)

Nor is the point of this book to fall into the same trap of cherry-picking the data to convince you that low-carb, high-fat diets are always bad and everyone should eat high-carb, low-fat diets. Nor is the point of this book to sell you on any other specific diet as being superior to low-carb, high-fat diets.

The point of this book is to help us all—as a society desperately in need of real solutions to improve our health and body composition—to move beyond the pseudoscientific villainization of carbohydrates to a rational and science-based approach to eating and health that is consistent with the entire body of scientific evidence and the experience of healthy humans.

We have personally witnessed far too many people who have been low-carb for years, who have gained nothing but a slower metabolism and an even fatter body, and are now dealing with fatigue, hypothyroidism, amenorrhea, low testosterone, and countless other health-related problems.

Having said that, if you are on a low-carb diet and you're getting the results you're after, this book is likely not for you. We have no desire to convince you to get off your low-carb diet, or to convince you that your diet is unhealthy or wrong in any way. We wish you the best, and we hope you will be blessed with continued good health!

On the other hand, if you're someone who is struggling on a low-carb diet, or perhaps considering yet another stint at low-carb dieting despite numerous previous failures, this book is for you. Ultimately, the purpose of this book is to help you break free of low-carb myths that are insidiously damaging your health and your psychological relationship with food, and to bring greater balance, vitality, and health into your life.

- If you are someone who has been avoiding carbohydrates for years and now find yourself dealing with various unexplained symptoms and health struggles, this book is for you.
- If you are someone who has been trying to lose fat or build muscle, you have been talked into adopting a low-carb diet, and the results you were promised haven't materialized, this book is for you.
- If you've been on a low-carb diet and you're now dealing with symptoms you and your doctor can't explain—perhaps things like fatigue, hypothyroidism/slow metabolic rate, stalled fat loss—this book is for you.
- If you are an athlete and have been trying to reduce your carbohydrate intake and increase your fat consumption so that you could become a "fat-burning machine" with "unlimited energy," but have instead found anxiety, sleeplessness, fatigue, and declining performance, this book is for you.
- If you are afraid of eating carbohydrates and sugars (and you habitually eat a fat-rich diet while pushing aside carbohydrate-rich foods) because you've been taught to believe things like "fats don't make you fat—carbs do" or "carbs spike insulin, which makes you fat" or "carbs cause diabetes," this book is for you.

The practical step of this book is a simple one: If you've been restricting carbohydrates and you're experiencing low energy, a slow metabolism, poor performance, fatigue, or other hormonal problems, just STOP!

Stop operating on false and unscientific beliefs about carbohydrates and stop restricting your carbohydrate intake. Stop trying to fight against your carbohydrate cravings. Stop beating yourself up with guilt every time you give in to the cravings. Most important is to *start* eating ample whole-food carbs again. Do it. You will feel better: today, tomorrow, and years from now.

Well, the practical steps to take are that simple. But getting to the point where you can actually *do* that—without guilt, self-flagellation, or fears of the carbohydrates turning into fat or making you a diabetic—is another story. Unfortunately, for most people who are operating on false and unscientific beliefs about carbohydrates/sugar/insulin, the only way to get past their "carbophobia" is through *knowledge*—through in-depth scientific understanding of the truth about how carbohydrates/sugar/insulin *really* affect our bodies.

Thus, this book is designed with one primary purpose: to debunk unscientific low-carb dogmas, which have been harming your health and quality of life, and thus allow you to liberate yourself from chronic low-carb dieting, to eat carbs again, and enjoy better health, a healthier psychological relationship with food, a better body, and a better quality of life, and to show you the real principles that matter when it comes to optimal health and body composition.

Get ready to explore radical new nutrition concepts unlike anything you've seen before and unlearn everything you thought you knew about carbohydrates.

You're about to discover:

- Why carbohydrates are not the disease- and obesity-inducing devils many popular low-carb gurus would like to have you believe, and why having ample amounts of the right kinds of carbohydrates is actually essential to your anti-aging, performance, health, and fat loss goals.
- That there is no body of well-controlled scientific studies that demonstrate that low-carb diets are superior for health, for performance, or for fat loss.
- Why wiring your body to "fat-burning" mode actually does not help you burn more fat on your body, and why many "fat-burning" diets are pure snake oil that will generally move you in the opposite direction of your health and fat loss goals.
- Why eating carbohydrates—and even sugar—is *not* the cause of type II diabetes, as most people believe.
- Why the Carbohydrate Theory of Obesity (the idea that carbs spike insulin, which makes us fat) is wrong on virtually every

level—which is why virtually no obesity scientist on the planet subscribes to this theory commonly promoted by low-carb diet gurus.

- That our Paleolithic ancestors certainly did not universally eat low-carb diets, as most low-carb Paleo advocates tell us.
- That the idea that burning fat or ketones for fuel instead of carbohydrates is going to lead athletes into superhuman performance is ridiculous and completely contradicted by the scientific evidence.
- Why fat is most definitely *not* our body's preferred fuel source or preferred way of operating.
- Why having a "fat-burning metabolism" from eating a high-fat, low-carb diet absolutely does not lead to *any* advantage for virtually *anything*—not health, not anti-aging, not exercise performance, and not fat loss.
- Finally, we'll show you the *real* nutritional factors that dictate how fat or lean you are (hint: it has little or nothing to do with the carbohydrate-to-fat ratio of your diet).

In short, what we're about to show you is why nearly every single claim made by low-carb diet advocates is at odds with the overall body of scientific evidence.

To be clear, this is definitely *not* to say that we disagree with everything promoted by most low-carb Paleo gurus. The Paleo movement has shown us some very valuable things: that there is indeed value in eating a whole-foods diet (both for health and body composition); that processed foods—including low-fat foods rich in refined sugars and grains—can be bad for us; that there is value in eating a high-protein diet; and that dietary fat and dietary cholesterol are not evil villains that should be avoided at all costs. Even more important, current Paleo writers have pointed out—through the lens of our evolutionary needs—the importance of proper sleep, exercise, family connections, and exposure to nature. These are great points for improving health and are at least as important as one's diet. **On all of these issues, we are in agreement with the low-carb Paleo advocates.**

Where many in the Paleo movement got it wrong was by accepting, with minimal scientific evidence, that humans are evolutionarily designed for low-carb diets, that eating carbohydrates is bad for us, and, in general, conflating the "Paleo diet" with the concept of low-carb dieting. This view (which is accepted by a few and challenged by most in the academic world) is not only an unscientific view, but it's also a dangerous one since many people who adopt low-carb diets consequently suffer from physical and psychological issues like hypothyroidism, anxiety, depression, fatigue, and insomnia. (To their credit, some thought leaders in the Paleo community—such as Chris Kresser, Paul Jaminet, and Robb Wolf—have evolved their thinking on carbohydrates tremendously over the last few years. We applaud these authors for their work, and our hope is that this book will inspire similar evolution in the thinking around carbohydrates in the more hardline anti-carbohydrate circles.)

Simply put, there is no body of scientific evidence that tells us that eating a low-carb, high-fat diet is the healthiest diet, no body of scientific evidence that suggests that eating a low-carb diet is either necessary or superior for fat loss, and no indication from examining traditional human populations that this is the diet of our ancestors or the optimal human diet.

It is an indisputable fact that it is possible for one to lose just as much weight and improve one's health from eating an extreme high-carb vegan diet as from an ultra-low-carb diet. This simple fact alone should tell you that there is far more to the story of good health and leanness than the proportion of your diet that you get from fat or carbohydrate.

It is impossible to account for the basic and indisputable fact that both vegans (who, in some cases, eat well over 600 or 800 grams of carbohydrate per day) can be just as lean and healthy as low-carbers (or leaner and healthier) who eat a mostly carnivorous diet while limiting carbohydrates below 75 grams per day. (Likewise, if you are a vegan who believes that one should eat only plant foods and that both animal fats and proteins are bad for us, it is impossible to account for the phenomenon that low-carbers eating diets composed almost entirely of protein and fat could be healthy and lean.) The reality is that there are millions of people eating diets of wildly different macronutrient ratios—from almost completely carnivorous low-carb diets to fruitarians eating basically nothing but sugar all day—who exhibit leanness and good health.

What that fact should tell anyone who is paying attention is that the answer to better health and fat loss isn't found in jettisoning one specific macronutrient from your diet. The answer isn't low-fat diets, low-protein vegan diets, or low-carb diets.

It should also tell you that all nutrition paradigms that promote the idea of a magical macronutrient ratio (whether the 80-10-10 fruitarians who eat 80% of their diet from carbohydrates or the low-carb ketogenic dieters who advocate that everyone should be eating a diet of 60-80% fat) are fundamentally misguided. The answer to the optimal diet is not in the macronutrients.

As explained in the beginning of this introduction, all macronutrients can be "scientifically proven to be bad for us." But at the same time, we will show you in this book that diets rich in any of the three macronutrients (or any combination of them) are all conducive to good health and a lean body.

In some ways, this book will debunk not only the notion that low-carb eating is the one true path to health and leanness, but also (indirectly) the notion that veganism or low-fat diets are the one true path as well. The reality is that good health and fat loss can be effectively achieved on a wide range of macronutrient ratios—from low carb to high carb and low fat to high fat. But, we must also recognize that *poor* health can be achieved with all these different approaches as well.

In addition to debunking the notion that carbohydrates are the cause of sickness and disease and that eating low-carb is the solution, this book will also show you the blueprint to the real nutritional factors that control your health and fat loss destiny. We will not be suggesting any specific diet to you as being superior to the low-carb, high-fat diet, nor will we suggest that there is some magical proportion of carbohydrates versus fat in the diet that will grant you incredible benefits.

There are other, far more important factors that dictate one's health and fat loss than how much fat or carbohydrate you eat each day. We will show you exactly what those factors are and provide you the blueprint for an optimal fat-loss diet. But let us emphasize that these are *principles,* and **there is a wide range of macronutrient profiles that you are free to experiment with to find your best health**.

You have a right to good health, physical and mental well-being, energy levels to achieve your goals, and freedom from worrying every day about what you eat. Before you give up that right by believing in those who would frighten you away from one food or another, please read on discover the *real* factors that determine your health and fat loss destiny.

Chapter 1: The Five Foundational Myths of Low-Carb Diet Dogma

In the 1980s and 1990s, health authorities told us that dietary fat was to blame for much of the nation's poor health, including rising rates of heart disease, diabetes, and obesity. This was the rise of the low-fat era, which was supposed to fix the obesity and heart disease epidemic in the United States.

The problem, however, is that for the next couple of decades, rates of obesity and diabetes continued to increase just as they had been doing before that.

Some people made this simple observation and theorized, "Well, low-fat didn't stop the obesity epidemic—people kept on getting fatter and having worse health. So maybe we had it wrong all along—maybe it's actually *carbs*, not fat, that are to blame for these problems."

And this makes some sense in that context, since the low-fat movement appeared to not only fail to reverse rising rates of obesity, but actually coincided with the worsening of the obesity epidemic. Based on that observation, it seemed reasonable to deduce that maybe carbs and sugar were the real problem.

Thus, the modern low-carb movement was born. Dozens of self-proclaimed health gurus became popular by telling the world that the low-fat diet had failed us all, and the *real reason we were fat and unhealthy was due to carbohydrates and insulin levels.*

But there was just one little problem with this theory...

WE NEVER ACTUALLY DID LOWER OUR FAT INTAKE!

In fact, the average fat intake has steadily climbed over the last 100 years. There was *never*—we repeat, *never*—a period in our history where hordes of people started eating low-fat diets and continued to become more obese. In fact, the research very clearly shows that those who actually do adhere to low-fat diets *do* indeed lose weight and improve their health. But as a society, we most definitely did *not* adopt low-fat diets.[3] [4]

Consider what the head of Yale's Prevention Research Center, David Katz, MD, has to say on the matter:

> "...the advice we got decades ago to cut dietary fat was never intended as advice to eat low-fat, high-starch, high-sugar cookies. **When the advice to cut fat was first provided, there was no such thing as highly processed, low-fat junk food.** The food industry exploited the advice and invented low-fat junk food to take advantage of it... The advice to cut fat was intended to direct us to the naturally low-fat foods that existed at the time, namely vegetables, fruits, beans, lentils, whole grains, and lean meats. ... **Studies that have looked at cutting fat by eating more naturally low-fat plant foods have, in fact, shown astonishing benefit—such as the reversal of coronary atherosclerosis, the prevention of heart attacks, and the favorable modification of gene expression... But that hypothesis was never tested at the population level. At the population level, we asked this: what will happen when Big Food takes advantage of the advice to reduce fat intake by inventing a whole new variety of junk food, and we all pretend that's what we thought the advice meant all along and eat a whole lot of that starchy, sugary junk and never actually reduce our**

3 http://wholehealthsource.blogspot.com/2012/0

3 http://www.ncbi.nlm.nih.gov/pubmed/88198919/more-thoughts-on-macronutrient-trends.html

4 http://www.cdc.gov/nchs/nhanes.htm

> **fat intake, either? I trust no one is too surprised with the answer: we will get fatter and sicker."**[5]

Thus, the notion commonly heard from low-carb gurus that the low-fat era consisted of millions of people adopting low-fat diets and getting fatter in the process is simply wrong. This notion completely ignores the facts of what really took place and ignores the scientific data that we have regarding people who do adopt whole-food-based, low-fat diets.

In the world of formal debating, this is known as the straw man fallacy, which is defined as ignoring the actual position/data and setting up a misrepresented or distorted version of that position in its place. That is exactly what low-carb gurus have done—their entire paradigm is built on top of a giant straw man.

We, as a nation, never actually lowered our dietary fat intake. The way things actually went down went something like this:

1) We were eating a high-fat diet prior to, and during, the initial stages of the obesity epidemic.
2) Then, researchers suggested that the high-fat diet may be a big reason why we were becoming fat and diabetic.
3) **Then, the low-fat era came into being, and during this time, we *kept our fat intake just as high,* and we simply added a bunch of refined grains, refined oils, and refined sugars *on top of* our normal high-fat diet.**

There were numerous other subtle shifts during this span as well. For example, we shifted away from using animal fats, and the use of vegetable oils and trans fats skyrocketed. Consumption of whole potatoes decreased dramatically while intake of fried potatoes skyrocketed. We added white flour and corn products in large amounts. And consumption of both refined grains and sugars increased by huge amounts on top of our already high-fat diets. Note also that low-carb gurus frequently like to distort the simple fact that we never lowered our fat intake by using misleading statistics, like the percentage of fat in the US diet. The *percentage* of fat in the diet did indeed decrease slightly from 37% fat to 33% fat. However, this does *not*—as they try to imply—mean that our actual fat consumption went

5 http://www.huffingtonpost.com/david-katz-md/diet-and-nutrition_b_4755777.html

down. What actually happened is that overall calories in the diet *increased* (by about 350 calories per day since 1970), and the additional calories were primarily from refined grain and sugar products. **Hence, the *percentage* of fat of the total calories decreased, but our *actual* fat consumption stayed just as high as it was before.** In fact, during the span from 1970 until present day, 65% of that increase in calories is from refined grain and sugar products and 24% is from fat. So our consumption of fat has actually *increased,* not decreased, *both since the start of the obesity epidemic and on the longer timeline of the last century.* If we look at macronutrient trends since 1909, the only macronutrient that *has* increased significantly over the last century is fat.[6]

So the notion that our country was getting fatter while we were all eating low-fat diets is false. We were getting fatter while eating high-fat (and high-refined-carbohydrate) diets, while health authorities were screaming at us to lower our fat intake, and we never really listened. In fact, not only did we not listen to the recommendations and lower our fat intake, but we actually *increased* our total calorie intake by several hundred calories and slightly *increased* our absolute fat intake in the process.

The result of all this: The United States continued its dominant reign as the fattest and most degenerative-disease-ridden population the world has ever known.

The reason the obesity epidemic kept on getting worse was never that the advice to eat a low-fat, plant-based diet was so flawed—it was the failure of the American public to actually follow the advice! The problem was the failure of the American people to lower their intake of fatty foods and adopt lower-fat diets in their place. The problem was that the food industry saw it as an opportunity to create all sorts of new "low-fat" and "non-fat" junk foods. The problem was that the American people—instead of lowering their fat intake and shifting to a more plant-based, low-fat diet—interpreted the recommendations as "only fat makes us fat" and saw it as an opportunity to eat those low-fat junk foods with impunity. Thus, they simply added a bunch of refined grain and sugar products (and even some fat) on top of their already high-fat diet.

---

6 http://wholehealthsource.blogspot.com/2012/09/more-thoughts-on-macronutrient-trends.html

Nonetheless, the low-carb movement was largely built around the notion that low-fat diets are a failure, that fat is not bad for us after all, and that carbohydrates/insulin/sugars are the real cause of obesity and most modern degenerative disease.

In fact, many low-carb Paleo advocates have actually taken things one step beyond just this. Not only do they claim—incorrectly—that we were getting fatter while eating low-fat diets, but on top of this myth, they have built another even more insidious myth. According to these low-carb advocates, not only were carbs making us sick and fat, and not only is fat not bad for us, but our health problems and obesity are in large part due to a *deficiency of dietary fat* because of the "low-fat craze that was sweeping the nation."[7] [8] [9] Then in a very everything-you-think-you-know-is-a-lie sort of move, they told us that the real problem is not only *not* too much fat in the diet, but too *little* fat! People are getting sick and fat, they told us, due to their cells being "starved" of fats! They typically use various scientific-sounding phrases to justify their notion that people's bodies are suffering because "fats are needed to synthesize hormones" or "your brain is made up of fats" or "cell membranes are composed of fats" (or various other claims about the roles of fat in the body). And many of these claims about fats are indeed accurate—fats do have very important functions in the body. The part that they got wrong isn't the role of fat in the body; it's the notion that lots of people (who in reality were mostly eating *high-fat* diets) were *deficient* in fats and needed to consume *more* fats in order to improve their health.

The low-carb advocates have since pulled off a rather remarkable feat—akin to the proverbial "selling ice to Eskimos": they have convinced a fat and sick population that had been world-renowned for eating one of the highest-fat diets on the planet that they were all actually eating a *low-fat* diet all along, and that the path to better health and a leaner body was actually an even *higher-fat* diet!

Fats, they told us, were what our bodies were meant to run on (we were all meant to be "fat burners" not "sugar burners") and are a magical source of energy that bestow upon its consumer all sorts of

---

7 http://www.more.com/health/healthy-eating/saturated-fat-good

8 http://greatist.com/health/saturated-fat-healthy

9 http://www.shape.com/healthy-eating/diet-tips/why-eating-man-may-be-best-womens-health

wonderful effects such as more energy, more stable energy (without the "crashes"), better hormonal health, a faster metabolism, a smarter brain, and, in general, that fats—not carbs—fuel superhuman performance.[10] [11] [12]

Thus, one myth has been built on top of another. To put all of this in visual form, it looks something like this:

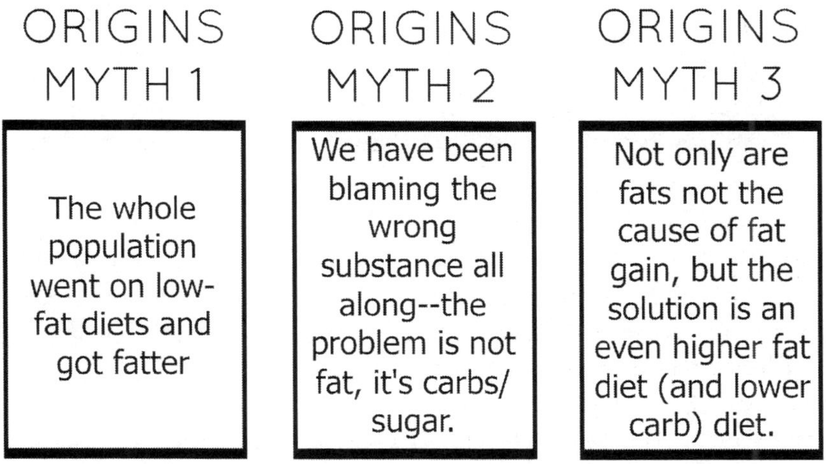

To be clear, all three of these notions are completely contradicted by the actual scientific data.

Nevertheless, out of these original myths, hundreds of other myths around carbohydrates, starches, sugars, and insulin have been perpetuated.

The internet and YouTube videos are chock full of warnings about how carbohydrates and sugar will damage your health and make you fat and diabetic. Here are some typical examples of the kinds of things you can expect to hear from low-carb diet advocates:

- "Carbs spike insulin, which makes you fat!"
- "Carbs spike insulin, which causes diabetes!"

---

10 http://articles.mercola.com/sites/articles/archive/2005/06/09/fatburn.aspx

11 http://fitness.mercola.com/sites/fitness/archive/2012/08/17/human-body-favors-fat-adaptation.aspx

12 http://www.marksdailyapple.com/what-does-it-mean-to-be-fat-adapted/

- "Eating a low-carb diet turns you into a fat-burning machine—which means instead of burning sugar, you're burning fat—and that will make you lean in no time!"
- "Fructose is toxic and damages your liver like alcohol!"
- "If you eat fat instead of carbs and avoid these insulin spikes, your body can't get fat. Insulin is the fat-storing hormone, so if you don't spike it, your body won't get fat."
- "It's not dietary fat that turns into body fat—it's sugar! Fat can't make you fat."
- "Carbs spike your blood sugar and then cause it to crash, which saps you of your energy! Burning fat for fuel gives you a stable source of energy without all the spikes and crashes."
- "We have 'essential fats' and 'essential amino acids' (i.e., proteins), but there's no such thing as 'essential carbohydrates'—therefore, carbs are less important."
- "Fat is the preferred source of fuel of your body, not carbs! You want to be a 'fat burner' not a 'sugar burner,' don't you?"
- "All the low-fat movement did was make us sicker and fatter."
- "Burning fat for fuel gives you a metabolic advantage and fuels superhuman athletic performance."
- "Our ancestors ate a low-carb diet because they didn't have grains, breads, and pastas—these are products of the agricultural revolution just 10,000 years ago. The diet of our ancestors was a low-carb diet since all they had available to them were things like animal foods, nuts/seeds, and green vegetables. We are not genetically adapted to eat a carbohydrate-based diet. That is why the Paleo diet is all about eating meat, green veggies/salads, and nuts and seeds—our ancestors didn't eat carbs, they ate a protein- and fat-based diet. Not like modern humans that eat tons of carbs."

And there are dozens more myths, which should remind us all that the internet is mostly uncensored, and the content is not peer reviewed or checked for accuracy. So don't believe everything you read or see on the internet.

In trying to sort out legitimate claims from pseudoscience, the challenge is to know where to begin, given the giant mess of carbohydrate myths that have been perpetuated for the past fifteen years. After analyzing the work of all the major low-carb gurus, we believe that there are really five foundational myths upon which the whole low-carb theory rests. These five foundational myths are:

1) "Carbs spike insulin, and insulin makes you fat!" This is known as the Carbohydrate/Insulin Theory of Obesity, which attempts to blame fat gain (and really the entire obesity epidemic) squarely on the shoulders of carbohydrates and sugars.
2) "Carbs spike insulin, which causes diabetes!" This is the ever-prevalent idea that it is the insulin spikes from consuming carbohydrates that cause insulin resistance.
3) "The Paleo diet is all about eating a low-carb, high-fat diet since it is a scientific fact that our ancestors didn't eat many carbs."
4) "Fats are the preferred source of fuel for the body, not carbs. Carbohydrates are not even 'essential' nutrients. We have 'essential fatty acids' (i.e., fats) and 'essential amino acids' (i.e., proteins), but there's no such thing as 'essential carbohydrates'—therefore, they are less important."
5) "Eating a low-carb diet turns you into a fat-burning machine. Instead of burning sugar, you're burning fat, which will make you lean in no time!" This is the idea that wiring your body to be more of a "fat burner" by eating a low-carb, high-fat diet results in burning off body fat.

These are the five foundational myths upon which the whole low-carb diet fad has been built. And as we are about to show you, every one of these is thoroughly unscientific, unsubstantiated by the data, and just plain wrong.

Chapter 2: The Carbohydrate Theory of Fat Gain - Wrong on Every Level

Perhaps the central pillar of the low-carb trend is the Carbohydrate Theory of Obesity. The Carbohydrate Theory of Obesity is essentially an attempt to blame fat gain, and the entire obesity epidemic, solely on carbohydrates and sugars. The basic premise is that when you eat carbohydrates, a hormonal state is created in your body that leads to fat storage.

Before we get into all the details of the theory—and why it's wrong—let's look at where this idea came from. The theory has gained prominence largely due to the work of a journalist by the name of Gary Taubes, who has written the books *Good Calories, Bad Calories* and *Why We Get Fat.*

Taubes' work is based on numerous scientific inaccuracies, omissions of data that conflict with his ideology, and countless instances of data cherry-picking. For anyone interested in seeing detailed analyses and deconstructions of Taubes' work, his many factual errors and misrepresentations have been outlined extensively by other authors such as obesity scientist Stephan Guyenet, PhD; physiology expert Lyle McDonald; researcher James Krieger; in an article by researcher George Bray, MD, published in *Obesity Reviews*; David Katz, MD; and by obesity scientist Yoni Freedhoff, MD. It's worth pointing out that many of these opposing opinions are from world-renowned MD and PhD researchers with extensive training related to nutrition, physiology, and research, while Mr. Taubes is a journalist with an engineering background.

To give a small sampling of the gist of what you will find in those articles:

- Here is a brief synopsis of Yoni Freedhoff, MD's analysis: **"Taubes seems to have decided to abandon journalistic and scientific integrity in place of observational data, straw men, and logical fallacy."**[13]
- From researcher George Bray: "**In developing his ideas about calories and obesity in *Good Calories, Bad Calories*, Taubes argues that obese individuals do not eat more than lean ones do. The data for his belief come from the Diet and Health Report prepared by the National Academy of Sciences. ... We now know that the data used in the Diet and Health Report were wrong** ..."[14]
- From James Krieger: "Supposedly Taubes did six years of research for this book, yet it took me only a few days of PubMed searches to find better research. Chapter 14 is more **an exercise in confirmation bias than true scientific inquiry.**"[15]
- David Katz, MD, notes that "Mr. Taubes and others like him—the iconoclasts out to save us from our confusion—worry the hell out of me" for the reasons he outlines in this stellar article.[16]

From physiology expert Lyle McDonald:

> **"A major part of Taubes' entire premise is based on a 1980 study that is incorrect. How come Taubes, in his '5 years of research,' wasn't able to realize that the self-reported food data in 1980 was wrong? It's 2009 and we know factually that the obese eat more than the lean. Yet somehow, Taubes was**

---

13 http://www.weightymatters.ca/2011/01/book-review-gary-taubes-why-we-get-fat.html

14 http://www.proteinpower.com/drmike/wp-content/uploads/2008/07/bray-review-of-gcbc.pdf

15 http://weightology.net/?p=265

16 http://www.huffingtonpost.com/david-katz-md/diet-and-nutrition_b_4755777.html

> **unable to come across that data point. And refuses to acknowledge it even now. What does that tell you about him and his agenda**?… Every aspect of his hypothesis is disproven by research, but he so carefully cherry-picks his data that he makes a convincing sounding argument that is just wrong. ... Bottom line: Taubes is wrong about everything he claims. **Yet in his '5 years of research' he seemed to never find the contradictory data. He pushed his agenda just as he claimed the anti-saturated fat people did."**[17]

Our purpose with this book is not to discredit Taubes' work specifically or point out the specific instances in which he has misrepresented the data in order to paint a picture of carbohydrates as being the cause of obesity. Many have already done that quite successfully.

More importantly, the notion of carbohydrates/sugar/insulin being "bad for us" or "making us fat" has gone mainstream, and it is now commonplace for the general public to believe that carbohydrates are a dietary scourge that is making us sick and fat. So rather than analyze Taubes' book, our purpose is to transparently address the scientific facts around carbohydrates and debunk the many myths that have been perpetuated about them.

Among these myths, the central myth upon which all the others depend is the Carbohydrate Theory of Obesity, or in simple terms, the "carbs make you fat" theory.

The theory that carbohydrates cause fat gain is built on three simple premises:

1) Insulin is the primary hormone that dictates how fat or lean we are.
2) Carbohydrates are the main substance that causes insulin levels to go up (both transiently and chronically).
3) Therefore, carbohydrates make you fat.

In other words, carbs cause your body to secrete insulin, which is a "fat-storing" hormone, and the more often you stimulate it (i.e., eat carbs), the fatter you get. Pretty simple and straightforward, right? And even pretty logical—if you are constantly boosting this hormone that

---

17 http://www.bodyrecomposition.com/fat-loss/insulin-levels-and-fat-loss-qa.html/

is causing you to store fat several times a day, that is probably what is making you fat… right?

Just so you know that we are not misrepresenting this theory or misstating the details, let's see how some leading low-carb gurus explain the Carbohydrate Theory of Fat Gain.

Gary Taubes defines the theory by saying:

> "This alternative hypothesis of obesity constitutes three distinct propositions. First, as I've said, is the basic proposition that obesity is caused by a regulatory defect in fat metabolism, and so a defect in the distribution of energy rather than an imbalance of energy intake and expenditure. The second is that insulin plays a primary role in this fattening process, and the compensatory behaviors of hunger and lethargy. The third is that **carbohydrates, and particularly refined carbohydrates—and perhaps the fructose content as well, and thus perhaps the amount of sugars consumed—are the prime suspects in the chronic elevation of insulin; hence, they are the ultimate cause of common obesity."** [18]

To put all this pseudoscientific nonsense in jargon-free language, he's simply saying:

1) Fat gain isn't actually caused by an imbalance of taking in more calories than you're burning—rather, it is because something is causing more of the calories to turn into body fat.
2) The key factor that causes all these calories to be turned into body fat is insulin.

Note: After saying that the reason people get fat is not due to overconsuming calories relative to how much they burn (#1 above), he then claims that insulin also happens to make you hungry (increases "calories in") and lazy (decreases "calories out"). This is a way to cover for himself in case his idea in #1 is proved false—if calories, not insulin, are the reason people become fat, then he can still claim that carbs are the reason people get fat by suggesting that they make you hungry and lazy, and thus, he could say "carbs make you fat by making you chronically consume more calories than you burn."

---

18 Taubes, G. Good Calories, Bad Calories.

3) Carbohydrates cause insulin spikes and are also the cause of chronically elevated insulin levels (i.e., insulin resistance). Therefore, carbohydrates are the primary cause of fat gain.

Andreas Eenfeldt, MD, the "Diet Doctor," says the same thing as Taubes in a much more direct and straightforward way:

"Carbohydrates → insulin → obesity

- **Thus more carbohydrates lead to more insulin, which leads to more fat accumulation.**

With more details, this can be written as follows:

Too many carbohydrates → pathologically high insulin levels → obesity

The opposite is the following:

Fewer carbs → lower insulin levels → loss of excess fat

- **Insulin is a fat-storing hormone. And the easiest way to increase your insulin levels is to eat more carbohydrates. The easiest way to lower insulin levels is to eat fewer carbohydrates."[19]**

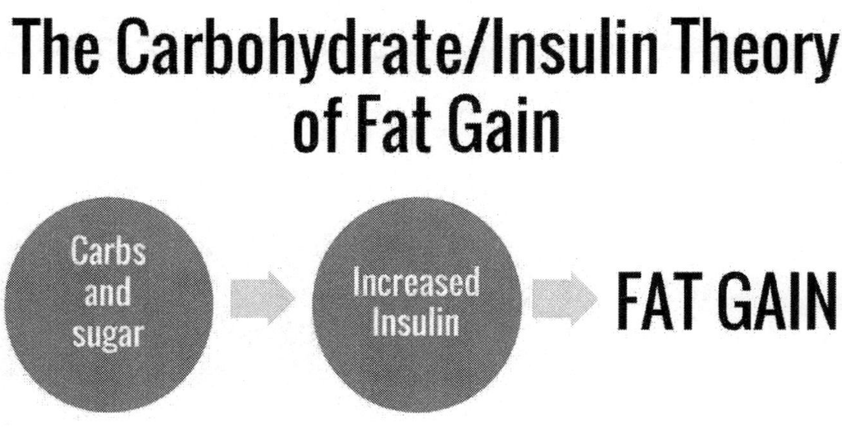

That's the Carbohydrate Theory of Obesity: you eat carbs, carbs raise insulin, and insulin creates fatness.

Good sounding theory, right?

---

19 http://www.dietdoctor.com/yes-a-low-carb-diet-greatly-lowers-your-insulin

The only problem is that there is a mountain of scientific evidence that completely contradicts it.

As a matter of fact, the Carbohydrate/Insulin Theory of Obesity had already been extensively studied by obesity scientists in the 1980s—decades prior to the low-carb diet fad of the 2000s. And after studying this specific issue thoroughly, virtually all obesity scientists on the planet then discarded the theory because it fails to explain numerous observations about fat gain/obesity. [20]

Let's now go over exactly what those basic observations are.

---

20 http://wholehealthsource.blogspot.com/2011/08/carbohydrate-hypothesis-of-obesity.html

Debunking the Low-Carb Mythology Regarding Insulin and Body Fatness

The carbohydrate hypothesis of obesity didn't materialize out of thin air. In truth, it came out of four observations that genuinely appear to link higher levels of insulin with fat gain. These observations are:

1) Obese people frequently (but not always) have higher baseline levels of insulin.
2) Type I and type II diabetics—after losing the ability to produce insulin—frequently lose weight and become very lean (to the point of looking like they're wasting away), and they often gain weight after injecting insulin.
3) Type II diabetics who inject insulin sometimes become overweight.
4) People with insulinomas (insulin-producing tumors) often become ravenously hungry and obese if left untreated.

On the surface, these observations seem to be unequivocal proof that insulin is a major player in how fat or lean we are. But let's take a closer look at these four observations and see if that really holds true upon closer examination.

WHY DO OBESE PEOPLE USUALLY HAVE HIGHER LEVELS OF INSULIN?

First, let's look at #1—the idea that because obese people often have higher baseline levels of insulin, it means that fat gain is caused by those higher levels of insulin. It is true that, in general, insulin levels do parallel bodyweight, and the vast majority of the time, obese people do have higher baseline insulin levels. The only part that is not true is the causation—obesity is not caused by insulin resistance or higher levels of insulin. But the opposite is true—higher levels of body fat do induce insulin resistance, and thus, lead to higher baseline levels of insulin. This is a case of confusing correlation with causation.

Consider this quote from obesity researcher Stephan Guyenet:

> **"Manipulating insulin signaling can change fat mass, and obese people have higher insulin, so it must be involved in obesity, right?** Unfortunately, these arguments fall apart upon closer scrutiny, not because they're based on

> inaccurate observations, but because they're irrelevant to common obesity. In obesity as in most other conditions where insulin is high, elevated insulin is a symptom of insulin resistance, and the two occur in parallel. **The pancreas secretes more insulin because the tissues can't 'hear' it as well, so they need more of it to do the job. The more insulin resistance, the more insulin. The key point here is that elevated insulin in obesity is a compensatory response to insulin resistance, i.e., a reduced insulin signal.** The cells are not seeing more insulin signaling, because they're insulin resistant, so it makes no sense to invoke increased insulin action to explain common obesity."[21]

In other words, higher levels of insulin are a symptom of the metabolic dysfunction (i.e., insulin resistance) that tends to happen in obese people—it's not the cause of their obesity. This increase in insulin levels compensates for the underlying dysfunction (either completely or partially), and nutrients flow in and out of cells in much the same way that a healthy insulin-sensitive person would be responding to normal levels of insulin. Either way, the cell itself is, at best, seeing normal insulin signaling and, at worst, less-than-normal insulin signaling.

That last part—that the increase in insulin does not actually translate into the cells receiving higher levels of insulin--is critical. Why? Because the Carbohydrate Theory of Obesity is built on the premise that higher baseline levels of insulin actually make people fat by keeping fat trapped in cells and preventing it from being burned off.

This is significant because research has already shown that this is wrong—obese people with higher circulating levels of insulin do not have any deficit in the ability to burn fat due to their higher levels of insulin. The reason why insulin is elevated is precisely because their cells are insulin resistant due to their obesity—thus even with higher baseline levels of insulin, the cells are not actually receiving that signal, and thus, they release fat into the bloodstream just fine. In fact, there is a great deal of evidence showing that insulin is actually stimulated

---

21 http://wholehealthsource.blogspot.com/2011/08/carbohydrate-hypothesis-of-obesity.html

precisely because of such a large fat mass (i.e., being obese), constantly dumping fatty acids into the bloodstream. The body is doing its best to prevent excessive release of fatty acids from the cells, which would create toxic levels of fatty acids in the blood. We know this is true because overall fatty acid delivery and fat burning remain as high or even higher in obese people.

According to Guyenet:

> **"Obese people do not have a defect in the ability to release fat from fat cells and burn it, to the contrary. They release more fat from fat cells than lean people, and burn more of it."** [22] [23] [24] [25]

The people with the highest insulin levels actually tend to be even better at releasing fat from fat cells. They are more efficient "fat burners" even though they are obese! Higher levels of insulin in overweight people are not preventing their body fat from being burned off. So this whole notion that those who have chronically elevated levels of insulin are worse at burning fat, and therefore accumulate body fat, is clearly incorrect.

Simply put, insulin is not doing what low-carb gurus claim—it is not keeping fat trapped in fat cells and causing body fat accumulation.

For now, the important fact to realize is that insulin levels do indeed often parallel bodyweight, but this does not mean that insulin *causes* fat accumulation. What's really going on is that chronic overconsumption of calories drives body fat accumulation, and body fat accumulation itself (and chronic calorie overconsumption) is the major cause of insulin resistance. (This chain of causality will be discussed further in the chapter on insulin resistance.) In other words, the reason obese people have higher levels of insulin is not because they first had high insulin levels and then the insulin caused them to get fatter—it's because chronically overconsuming calories and piling on body fat made them insulin resistant, which in turn caused their insulin levels to go up.

---

22 http://wholehealthsource.blogspot.com/2011/08/carbohydrate-hypothesis-of-obesity.html

23 http://www.ncbi.nlm.nih.gov/pmc/articles/PMC303803/

24 http://www.ncbi.nlm.nih.gov/pubmed/5806343

25 http://www.ncbi.nlm.nih.gov/pubmed/8405696

So that takes care of observation #1—the fact that obesity is correlated with higher levels of insulin.

WHY DO DIABETICS WHO CANNOT PRODUCE INSULIN LOSE WEIGHT?

Now, we still have a few other observations to deal with regarding the correlation between insulin and body fatness. Let's look at #2—the observation that type I and type II diabetics who have lost the ability to produce insulin frequently lose weight and become very lean (to the point of looking like they're wasting away) and often gain weight after injecting insulin.

Just as with the apparent link we explored above between obesity and insulin resistance, here too we appear to have a clear link between high levels of insulin and being fat, and low levels of insulin and being lean. So if having the inability to produce insulin leads to leanness and having tons of insulin (from an insulin-producing tumor) leads to being fat, how could it be possible that insulin is not the cause of fat gain?

Well, the answer to this question requires that we go into a bit of physiology.

The first and most important thing we need to understand here is that insulin is indeed required for fat storage. However, **insulin does not *regulate* fat storage**.

This is a critical distinction. **Insulin is needed for the actual biochemical process of fat storage, but it is not the controller that dictates how much fat is stored or burned off.**

Without legs, it's impossible to run. But simply having legs does not dictate how far one runs (or doesn't run) each day. In the same way, there is a difference between something that is *required* for fat storage versus something that *regulates* fat storage. This is a critical distinction that is simply not understood by many advocates of low-carb diets.

Insulin is required for fat storage, but the amount of insulin in the body is not the factor responsible for dictating whether any normal healthy person is lean or fat.

Put more simply: If you do not have a pancreas or your pancreas has lost the ability to produce insulin (from type I diabetes or progressed type II diabetes), you will literally be unable to store fat. Sounds good, right? Maybe some low-carb advocates who think that the lower insulin, the better, might be tempted to think, "We should all be so lucky as to not have any insulin—then none of us would ever be able to get fat!" Right? Well, not so fast. What happens when you do not have insulin is that not only can't you store fat, but you also don't have insulin to drive glucose and protein into cells efficiently, and you have unrestrained lipolysis (i.e., fat cells dumping fats into the bloodstream beyond the body's ability to burn them off) and unrestrained gluconeogenesis (excessive production of glucose by the liver--raising blood sugar levels), and as a result, your muscles and organs waste away and, eventually, you die. The lack of insulin is not a state of health—it's a pathological disease state, and just as a non-functional pancreas that doesn't produce insulin causes leanness, so too can anorexia, malnutrition, and famine cause leanness. We can assure you, type I diabetics feel a whole lot better when they are treated with insulin than when they are not.

When you do not have insulin, production of glucose by the liver is unrestrained (which is one of the major roles of insulin). So you have a situation where there are lots of glucose molecules constantly being dumped into your bloodstream by the liver, but instead of those nutrients getting into your cells where they can be used or stored for energy, a large portion of them are excreted in the urine. [26] (Diabetes mellitus actually means "sweet urine.") When glucose levels exceed a certain level, this maxes out the kidneys' ability for glucose reuptake and you get large amounts of sugar being urinated out. It's like trying to fill your tub with water when your drain plug doesn't hold. Again, this inability to regulate blood sugar due to lack of insulin is extremely damaging to the body. Thus, adding insulin to that system helps prevent the loss of large amounts of glucose per day—effectively increasing "calories in" potentially by hundreds of calories per day—and allows the fat cells to actually do their job. Now the person has the ability to store fat like a normal healthy person (instead of wasting away due to unrestrained lipolysis and the loss of hundreds of calories of glucose). Instead of peeing out hundreds of calories each day, those vital nutrients can be used by the cells. In this case, injecting insulin takes someone out of a pathological disease state and returns them to a state of relatively normal healthy physiology and normal body fatness (instead of wasting away). Thus, diabetic patients often gain some fat—typically the amount a normal person would carry—as they get healthier from the insulin treatments. This same scenario happens with

---

26 http://carbsanity.blogspot.com/2013/10/the-cause-of-hyperglycemia-in-type-2.html

progressed type II diabetics who have decreased pancreatic function—they are essentially the same as type I diabetics in this regard.

The point here is that injecting insulin isn't causing them to become fat—it's causing them to be able to function like a normal healthy person who has a functional pancreas.

That takes care of why diabetics can waste away in the absence of insulin, and why, after injecting insulin, they go from a state of wasting to storing fat like a normal healthy person.

WHY DOES INJECTED INSULIN CAUSE WEIGHT GAIN IN DIABETICS, AND WHY DO INSULIN-PRODUCING TUMORS CAUSE WEIGHT GAIN?

You might be thinking now about the last couple of those four observations:

It is true that type II diabetics who inject insulin sometimes become overweight. Likewise, it is also true that insulin-producing cancers (insulinomas) can cause people to become overweight or obese.

This seems to be the most conclusive evidence that higher levels of insulin do indeed cause fat gain. Except for just a couple of things…

First, in humans, we don't just secrete insulin by itself; we secrete insulin and a satiety hormone called amylin together. This is why carbohydrate-containing meals (that do spike insulin) have been shown not to cause hunger and further consumption of calories. Injecting insulin (without amylin) does not adequately mimic normal human physiology. When injected insulin is administered along with amylin to diabetics, it actually causes weight loss.[27] [28] [29] Thus, it is rather nonsensical to extrapolate from the effects of pure insulin injections in diabetics to healthy persons eating carbohydrates. They are totally different states of physiology.

Second, and most important, we must remember what insulin's role in the body actually is—keeping the appropriate balance of nutrients in the blood so that nutrients can be delivered to where they need to go. Now, normally, insulin is secreted by the body in direct proportion to the nutrients present in the blood—that is, if nutrients are elevated a very small amount, you only get a very small amount of insulin, and if you consume huge amounts of food, you get much more insulin—in exactly the amount necessary to bring blood nutrients back down to baseline.

So given that function of insulin, what happens when you have a situation where the dose of insulin is not in perfect proportion to the amount of nutrients in the blood? Say, if you are a diabetic and you

---

27 http://www.ncbi.nlm.nih.gov/pubmed/16935845

28 http://www.ncbi.nlm.nih.gov/pubmed/12610038

29 http://www.ncbi.nlm.nih.gov/pubmed/11919132

inject too much insulin, or if you have a tumor that is producing lots of insulin well beyond any elevation in blood sugar?

Well, it doesn't just lower blood sugar back to the normal baseline level (like it would in any normal, non-diseased person), but it actually creates excessively low blood sugar—as in hypoglycemia.

What happens when you have low blood sugar?

Well, hypoglycemia is a potent trigger for food intake. It causes a major hormonal response—known as the "counter-regulatory response"—which is a desperate effort by the brain to avoid hypoglycemic coma and death. This response triggers epinephrine and glucagon release, resulting in ravenous hunger in a frantic effort to raise circulating glucose levels. [30] When this happens repeatedly, the predictable result is overconsumption of calories and fat gain.

So, yes, excessively large doses of insulin beyond the body's actual need for insulin—either from an insulin injection or a tumor that produces insulin—can cause increased fat accumulation as a result of hypoglycemia and the body's counterregulatory response that creates ravenous hunger and calorie overconsumption. **But again, this has no relevance to normal human physiology and common obesity.**

So here's where insulin can indeed make people gain lots of fat:

- The insulin has to be a sufficiently large dose to induce hypoglycemia, which means it has to be a supraphysiological dose (a dose well beyond the body's normal production of insulin) that is well in excess of the body's actual need for insulin.
- That hypoglycemia-inducing, supraphysiological dose of insulin has to also be administered without insulin's normal partner hormone amylin—an appetite suppressing hormone—which is always secreted with insulin in any normal person.

Thus, for anyone trying to implicate insulin in fat gain in normal people, there are just a couple of little problems: These two scenarios only happen if you inject hypoglycemia-inducing amounts of insulin (which virtually never happens in any normal body) and without amylin (which never happens in any normal body).

30 http://wholehealthsource.blogspot.com/2012/01/insulin-and-obesity-another-nail-in.html

Also worth noting is that an additional cause of obesity in diabetics is the preponderance of associated health problems often caused by diabetes. A high proportion of diabetic patients have cardiac and peripheral vascular disease, retinal dysfunction, and other conditions that limit exercise and activity. In those patients with difficulty maintaining normal blood glucose levels due to compliance issues, "brittle" diabetes, or the effects of other medications, the large shifts in glucose levels can lead to a myriad of eating difficulties. The challenges of poor glucose control, associated health problems, and lowered physical activity levels lead to weight gain and a cycle of poor health. This unfortunately common scenario is NOT a valid comparison model for non-diabetic, relatively healthy people trying to understand the healthiest way to eat.

In other words, the problem with trying to relate the effect of injected insulin, as learned from studies on diabetes, to common overweight and obesity is that there is essentially no relevance whatsoever. This would be the equivalent of saying, "injecting testosterone (i.e., steroids) can be harmful; therefore, testosterone is a 'bad hormone,' and we should all be trying to lower our own body's production of testosterone as much as possible." Clearly that is a ridiculous conclusion, as lowering our body's own production of testosterone would be a bad thing, leading to declining health. Yet, the people who try to liken the effects of insulin injections or insulin-producing tumors to what is happening in a normal healthy person's body are making a similarly illogical statement.

Overweight and obese people have a state of physiology (insulin resistance) that is characterized by <u>decreased insulin signaling</u> at the cell level and <u>high</u> blood sugar (<u>hyper</u>glycemia). In contrast, the situation where injected insulin (or insulinomas) causes fat gain is in the context of massively <u>increased insulin signaling</u> (due to excess insulin beyond the body's needs) and <u>low</u> blood sugar (<u>hypo</u>glycemia).

In common obesity, **cells are not receiving adequate amounts of insulin to lower blood sugar even to normal baseline levels, let alone to levels low enough to induce hypoglycemia and a counterregulatory response**. To the contrary, obese people typically have high blood sugar and high blood free fatty acids! Therefore, the hypoglycemia counterregulatory response (seen in those with insulin-producing tumors and those injecting insulin) doesn't bear resemblance to common overweight and obesity. Thus, it makes no sense to invoke insulin to explain overweight and obesity in normal people.

As Guyenet states:

"The effects of insulin in the context of diabetes, insulinoma, and hypoglycemia are easily explained and bear little relevance to normal physiology."[31]

<u>Summary of the Obesity-Insulin Connection:</u>

- The observation that obesity and insulin levels parallel one another is not due to a causal relationship where insulin resistance is causing body fat accumulation. Rather, it is explained by the fact that obesity and diabetes are both characterized by the same factor—chronic caloric excess. Moreover, the causation is actually the opposite of what low-carb gurus claim—the real cause is that body fat accumulation tends to cause insulin resistance, not the other way around.
- Type I diabetics frequently go from a wasting condition to recovering normal levels of body fat after starting insulin therapy. This is because without insulin, they do not have the ability to store fat (or use nutrients very well), and thus they enter a chronic state of wasting away. Insulin allows them to recover relatively normal healthy physiology by allowing the cells to take in and store energy (thus preventing hundreds of calories from being urinated out), and this change in the calories in, calories out equation typically causes them to go from a state of wasting back to a normal healthy level of body fatness. (The same is true for type II diabetics for whom the disease has progressed far enough that the pancreas is no longer producing sufficient insulin—it creates a similar situation to type I diabetics, and injecting insulin has the same effects.) The absence of any other hormone or enzyme or component of the cell involved in fat storage would also cause this same wasting effect that the absence of insulin does—things like removing the ribosomes or DNA polymerase from fat cells, for example. And putting those vital components of the cell back in would similarly result in the ability to store fat like a normal healthy

---

31 http://wholehealthsource.blogspot.com/2012/01/insulin-and-obesity-another-nail-in.html

person. This is precisely what insulin is doing. The absence of insulin is not a condition of healthy fat loss; it is a pathological disease state.

- Type II diabetics who inject insulin and those with insulin-producing tumors often become fat. These people get fat to the degree that they have an amount of insulin that creates hypoglycemic episodes. The insulin isn't causing fat gain due to insulin preventing fat burning or increasing fat storage, but rather due to the fact that insulin is being produced in supraphysiological doses (i.e., would never occur in a normal overweight person) that are creating hypoglycemia and the counterregulatory response. This physiology never occurs in any normal person who does not inject insulin or have an insulin-producing tumor, and thus has zero relevance to common overweight and obesity.

The four observations about insulin and body fatness made by the low-carb gurus fail to suggest that elevated insulin has any relevance to fat gain in normal people.

With the notion that insulin is the cause of fat gain now debunked, let's take a more direct look at the notion that carbohydrates make us fat.

Why the Carbohydrate Hypothesis of Fat Gain Is Wrong

The Carbohydrate Hypothesis of Fat Gain states that ingestion of carbohydrates stimulates insulin, which causes increased rates of fat storage. The result is that, theoretically, if two people were eating the same number of calories per day but one was eating low carb and the other was not, the "carb eater" would gain more fat. The non-carb eater would not stimulate insulin and therefore could eat and eat without gaining fat.

When the theory is described in these simple terms, it sounds ridiculous (because it is). However, there seems to be something deeply alluring about being able to consume however much we want with impunity, so long as we avoid eating one particular kind of thing (i.e., "It's not the overall *food* you're eating that's making you fat; it's only the fat-storing hormone insulin that's coming from those evil carbohydrates!"). Thus, many people have been convinced that this theory is true and have changed their entire diet in hopes of eating all they want and not gaining fat.

The good news is that this theory is a relatively easy one to prove or disprove. We can test it with a few simple questions:

1) Does increasing or decreasing insulin levels within the normal physiological range (i.e., without inducing hypoglycemia) change how fast we gain or lose fat? More specifically, do studies show that higher levels of insulin cause more body fat accumulation as low-carb gurus claim?
2) Does insulin make you hungry and lazy? In other words, does insulin alter the calories in/calories out equation, as low-carb gurus claim? Does insulin cause decreased calorie expenditure (through fatigue or decreased metabolic rate) and increased calorie intake (through appetite/hunger stimulation) like Gary Taubes' Insulin Theory of Obesity suggests?
3) Do carbohydrates "turn into fat" as many low-carb advocates suggest (e.g., "fat doesn't make you fat—sugar does!")? After all, for insulin-spiking carbohydrates to be the cause of fatness, those carbohydrates have to be turned into fat before being stored as body fat. Carbs cannot work to cause fat gain simply by keeping fat trapped in fat cells—that could only cause you

to maintain your current level of body fatness. In order to actually accumulate body fat, something—some kind of calories—has to be getting turned into fat and piled on top of existing amounts of body fat. Where is that coming from?

4) Is the fat loss that is often seen on low-carb diets (e.g., low-carb Paleo) actually due to carbohydrate avoidance and lower levels of insulin? Or is it due to some confounding factor, like high protein intake or whole food intake—known factors that drive down total calorie consumption?
5) Do populations that eat more calories from carbohydrates have higher rates of obesity and overweight? If carbohydrates and insulin are the cause of fat gain, we should expect to see a significant correlation between populations that eat more carbohydrates and overall higher levels of body fat.

These questions allow us to directly test The Carbohydrate/Insulin Theory of Fat Gain. So here we go…

Insulin Does Not Cause Fat Gain, and Lowering Insulin Does Not Accelerate Fat Loss

If fat gain is caused by elevated levels of insulin, then interventions that suppress insulin should reliably prevent fat gain. Let's see if that's true.

The studies that have tested this hypothesis by lowering insulin levels either through diet, drugs, or genetic manipulation fail to show any fat loss effect.

One study placed two groups of overweight people on a low-calorie diet for eight weeks—one with the insulin-lowering drug diazoxide and one with a placebo. While diazoxide did indeed lower insulin levels, no differences in weight loss, fat loss, resting energy expenditure, or appetite were observed between the two groups.[32]

Many studies have used animal models that are genetically manipulated to maintain insulin sensitivity in response to obesity-inducing diets, which allows these mice to have exceptionally low insulin levels. These studies have proven over and over again that fat gain does not differ between animals that have high or low insulin levels—that is, they all get fat at the same rate. By knocking out various proteins and inflammatory signaling molecules (such as TNF-alpha, jun kinase 1 [JNK1], and inducible nitric oxide synthase [iNOS]), researchers can completely prevent the elevated insulin levels and insulin resistance that normally occurs during exposure to a fattening diet. Yet, these animals—despite much lower levels of insulin—get fat at roughly the same rate and, in some cases, actually gain ***more*** fat.[33] [34] [35]

When dogs are intentionally made obese on a fattening diet, they can be administered clonidine—a blood pressure drug that also acts to prevent insulin resistance and lower insulin levels—without any effect on the rate of fat gain. As in, dogs fed the diet with clonidine do indeed

---

32 Due A, et al. No effect of inhibition of insulin secretion by diazoxide on weight loss in hyperinsulinaemic obese subjects during an 8-week weight-loss diet. Diabetes, Obesity and Metabolism, Jul 2007; 9 (4): 566-574.

33 http://www.ncbi.nlm.nih.gov/pubmed/11590438

34 http://www.ncbi.nlm.nih.gov/pubmed/9335502

35 http://www.ncbi.nlm.nih.gov/pubmed/17983584

have lower insulin levels than dogs not taking clonidine, but they get fat at the exact same rate.[36]

If high levels of insulin are a major factor in obesity, one would expect to see elevated insulin in all, or virtually all, obese people. However, there is a subgroup of obese people who are considered "metabolically healthy obese people" and have normal fasting insulin and insulin sensitivity. In addition, there is a subset of lean people who have high insulin and low insulin sensitivity despite a normal fat mass (called "metabolically obese" people).[37] If insulin is *THE* cause—or even a primary cause—of fat gain, we should not have significant quantities of lean people with high insulin and fat people with low insulin. But we do.

These studies all demonstrate that insulin is not the major factor that determines how fat or lean we are. There is no body of peer-reviewed scientific studies that supports the idea that insulin causes people to be fat. Rather, the evidence is conclusive that insulin levels do not determine fatness.

Taubes and the rest of the low-carb gurus say that carbs and insulin are the culprits behind fat gain and obesity, and if you lower insulin levels, you have the recipe for a lean body. Yet when you actually examine well-controlled studies on the subject, they pretty much blow that idea to smithereens. They demonstrate that not only can insulin and body fatness be completely dissociated from one another, but they plainly show that raising or lowering insulin levels does not impact body fatness in any significant way.

If higher levels of insulin led to fat gain, this would be an incredibly easy thing to verify through research.

Thus, the simple fact that virtually every well-controlled study fails to detect such an effect makes it clear that insulin is not a major factor in fat gain or fat loss.

---

36 http://www.ncbi.nlm.nih.gov/pubmed/9931163

37 http://www.ncbi.nlm.nih.gov/pubmed/15181025

Even with All Their Carbohydrate Avoidance, Low-Carbers Are Still Spiking Insulin!

Virtually the entire rationale for eating low-carb is because of insulin. Low-carb advocates believe that insulin is the source of problems (fat gain, diabetes, etc.) and that insulin is increased by eating carbohydrates. "Carbs spike insulin, and these spikes of insulin make you fat and diabetic, so we should keep insulin low by avoiding carbohydrates." Thus, low-carb gurus (and many lay people) often *equate* carbohydrates with insulin—that is, we think of the presence or absence of insulin as directly proportional to the amount of carbohydrates in that meal.

This is fundamentally wrong!

If we look at a chart of the insulin index of certain foods, we find something remarkable. Many protein- and fat-containing foods—foods commonly advocated on low-carb diets with *the specific rationale that those foods are good because they keep insulin low*—actually increase insulin levels to a similar, and sometimes even greater, degree than many high-carbohydrate containing foods!

Numerous foods eaten on low-carb diets cause insulin spikes as massive as carbohydrate foods that the low-carbers commonly demonize on the basis that they stimulate insulin.

For example, beef and fish release as much insulin as brown rice. Beef, fish, and cheese actually release *more* insulin per calorie than pasta (white or brown) and porridge.[38]

Saturated fats like butter can even be insulinogenic—to the point where some low-carb gurus are concerned about it![39] Whey protein—a favorite of low-carb advocates—spikes insulin as much as white bread.[40] In general, meat spikes insulin as much or more than many common carbohydrate sources.

The whole point of eating low-carb was to avoid spiking insulin, and it doesn't even accomplish that!

*Side notes for nutrition geeks:

---

38 http://ajcn.nutrition.org/content/66/5/1264.abstract

39 http://livinlavidalowcarb.com/blog/does-butter-raise-insulin-and-make-you-fat-the-low-carb-experts-respond-to-this-claim/7573

40 http://suppversity.blogspot.com/2012/06/whey-more-insulinogenic-than-white.html

1) Many low-carb gurus still try to hold to their carbohydrate-insulin-fat gain theory dogmas even in the face of information like this that clearly destroys the very foundation of their belief system. They do so by trying to invoke the action of glucagon, suggesting that this opposes the effects of insulin, and therefore, even though high-protein meals boost insulin, the increase in glucagon cancels out the effects of insulin. Does this sound like dogmatic ideologues desperately trying to hold on to their belief system with stupid arguments? Good, because that's exactly what it is. Glucagon does indeed balance out blood sugar, preventing the hypoglycemia that would otherwise result, but in terms of fat metabolism, it absolutely does not oppose insulin.[41] Thus, this counterargument is bunk. Low-carbers, even after all their strict carbohydrate avoidance and ketogenic diets, *still* have lots of that "evil, fat-storing devil hormone" insulin in their system when they eat their low-carb meals.
2) It is not necessarily the case that overall average insulin levels throughout the day will be the same regardless of whether one eats a "low-carb" diet or a "high-carb" diet. This greatly depends on the specific types of foods one consumes. But in general, low-carb diets do tend to decrease insulin-producing foods, which is why low-carb diets tend to lower overall *average* insulin levels (as previously mentioned). Note, too, as we previously mentioned, that the decreased insulin levels do not mean anything significant, as they do not actually translate into fat loss.
3) Contrary to popular myth, eating fat with a carbohydrate-containing meal does *not* lower insulin levels from the meal—it actually *increases* insulin levels![42] Dr. William Davis, the author of the best seller *Wheat Belly,* actually has expressed concern about the insulin raising effects of *butter*, believe it or not.[43]

This is yet another deathblow to the foundations of low-carb dogma. Even the most basic of assumptions that low-carb dieting is

---

41 http://wholehealthsource.blogspot.com/2013/04/glucagon-dietary-protein-and-low.html

42 http://suppversity.blogspot.com/2014/09/the-pro-insulinogenic-activity-of.html

43 http://livinlavidalowcarb.com/blog/does-butter-raise-insulin-and-make-you-fat-the-low-carb-experts-respond-to-this-claim/7573

built on—that by avoiding carbohydrates, you will avoid elevating insulin and inhibiting fat burning—is wrong. Despite all their carbohydrate avoidance, low-carb dieters are *still* getting insulin spikes, and in some cases, just as massive or more massive insulin spikes on their low-carb diets.

Carbohydrates Do Not "Block" the Burning of Body Fat Any More than Protein or Fats Do

The typical low-carb guru spiel revolves around hormone-sensitive lipase (HSL), which is a key player in releasing fat from fat cells so it can be burned for energy. "Lipase" means "breaks down/releases fat," and the "hormone-sensitive" part means that in order for HSL to be activated, it requires the presence of certain hormones. Which ones? Well, basically the catecholamines, adrenaline and noradrenaline, activate HSL. Once the gurus explain to you that the key step to burning off all your body fat is by getting HSL activated through the release of adrenaline and noradrenaline, they'll go on to explain that it is insulin that is inhibiting HSL and therefore preventing you from being a "fat-burning machine." They then conclude, "Therefore, in order to burn off our body fat, we need stay in the fat-burning zone by avoiding carbohydrates since they spike insulin and shut down HSL."

There is a superficial logic to this: If insulin really is responsible for blocking the release of fat from fat cells, then how could you possibly expect to burn any fat off your body if you're always "spiking" your insulin levels by eating carbohydrates?

But there's just two parts of the equation that the low-carb gurus like to leave out:

- **Protein—as in meat, seafood, protein powder, etc.—also spikes insulin levels very significantly, as we've already seen.** Thus, protein also shuts down HSL and shifts the body away from the burning of body fat. Moreover, this simple physiological fact is conveniently left out by low-carb diet advocates who would like to have you believe that only carbohydrates can spike insulin levels. As mentioned above, the truth is that a high-protein low-carb meal can spike insulin to a degree that is on par with a carbohydrate meal.
- **Dietary fat, even though it doesn't spike insulin levels, also shuts down HSL!** Moreover, the inhibition of HSL seems to be particularly strong with saturated fats—the type of fats most commonly advocated by low-carb gurus. [44] Much more

44 http://www.ncbi.nlm.nih.gov/pubmed/3014093

> important than the inhibition of HSL, however, is the fact that most dietary fat consumed is directly stored as body fat. [45]

In addition, there is good research to show that even very tiny elevations in insulin can dramatically inhibit fat loss. This is in contrast to the typical low-carb guru assumption that lipolysis occurs in direct proportion to the level of insulin present. In fact, it is more a situation of any very tiny elevation in insulin will shut down body fat burning—that is, no massive insulin spike is necessary to create this effect. Thus, while eating typical low-carb, high-fat meals may not spike insulin as highly as a carbohydrate-rich meal, they do still elevate insulin enough to completely suppress body's fat burning. Moreover, they typically keep insulin elevated for longer than a low-fat, carbohydrate-rich meal. Therefore, the notion that avoiding a large spike of insulin from carbohydrates in order to have a more smooth elevation and decrease (i.e., more prolonged) rise and fall of insulin may very well be *worse* in terms of inhibiting body fat burning. According to Lyle McDonald, author of *The Ketogenic Diet*, "Even fasting insulin levels inhibit lipolysis by up to 50%, and even small increases essentially turn off lipolysis completely. Some could easily interpret this as meaning that "eating carbs stops fat loss." Or it might lead them to conclude that a carbohydrate-based diet would make fat loss impossible. Tangentially I'd note, and one weird little study supports this, that spiking insulin (and letting it crash back down) might be superior for fat loss than the standard strategy of trying to keep insulin low but stable all day long. The reason is that even tiny amounts of insulin block lipolysis, so if you keep insulin low but stable all day, you are effectively impairing lipolysis.[46]

So, eating typical low-carb meals *still* increases insulin levels enough to completely shut down lipolysis, and potentially, may even inhibit lipolysis *for longer periods of time* than carbohydrate-induced insulin spikes.

In other words, any time you eat *anything,* you're either shutting down the systems in your body that burn body fat, or in the case of ingesting dietary fat, you're directly storing more fat in your fat cells!

---

45 http://diabetes.diabetesjournals.org/content/56/1/168.full.pdf

46 http://www.bodyrecomposition.com/fat-loss/insulin-levels-and-fat-loss-qa.html/

Why? Because food signals to your body that it doesn't have to start dipping in to its own stored fuel or go into emergency stress mode and start cannibalizing its own tissue in order to survive!

Carbs, proteins, and fats all signal to the body that energy is abundant and there's no need to start cannibalizing its own tissues in order to function.

Ultimately, 500 calories of fat contribute to just as much fat getting locked away in your fat cells as 500 calories of carbohydrates do.

Any time you eat *anything*, you are either shutting down the burning of body fat (in the case of carbohydrate) or directly piling more fat into fat cells (in the case of eating fat).

At equivalent calories, you will store precisely the same amount of fat in your fat cells either way at the end of the day.

Do Carbs Make You Fat Because They Make You Hungry and Lazy?

The simple reality is that calories are king, and the presence or absence of insulin has essentially no relevance to fat loss or fat gain. The number of calories consumed and burned—not whether you're eating carbohydrates or not—determines how much fat is lost or gained.

Guyenet sums up this idea very efficiently: ***"There is no energy fairy."***[47] What does that mean? It means that in order for something to actually cause fat accumulation, it must increase "calories in" or decrease "calories out." Body fat is physical matter. Matter has to be made of something—it has to accumulate from *something*. This "fat-storing" hormone insulin isn't an energy fairy that can magically cause fat gain through its mere presence even when "calories in" do not exceed "calories out."

Moreover—and this is a key point—if calories in do exceed calories out, then why do we even need to invoke insulin as a way of explaining fat accumulation? In that case, the fat gain is caused by the excess of calories, not by the presence of insulin.

Thus, in order for carbohydrates (or insulin) to be considered a "cause" of fat gain, carbs (or insulin) would somehow have to create a calorie excess beyond the amount of calories being burned every day. Unless there is an energy fairy that can magically transcend basic laws of thermodynamics (and last we checked, there is not), it is not possible for insulin to cause fat accumulation in the absence of a caloric excess. Thus, to cause fat gain, insulin would have to do more than just "promote fat storage" or "block fat burning"—it would have to somehow either increase the amount of calories you eat each day (make you hungrier) or it would have to decrease caloric expenditure (make you lazy and not want to exercise).

Indeed, Gary Taubes is aware of this simple fact and theorized that insulin does indeed do exactly that:

---

47 http://wholehealthsource.blogspot.com/2011/08/carbohydrate-hypothesis-of-obesity.html

> **"...insulin plays a primary role in this fattening process, and the compensatory behaviors of hunger and lethargy."**[48]

Fortunately for us, this theory has been tested in numerous studies.

First, let's look at the idea that insulin increases hunger (i.e., food intake). Studies have found that when protein intake is kept the same, high- and low-carbohydrate meals, which vary in insulin response, do not cause different effects on satiety and subsequent food intake. [49] [50] [51] [52] **In fact, several of those studies show that high-carbohydrate meals result in greater satiety.** Moreover, if we look at protein—which, it bears repeating, also stimulates insulin release—satiety is positively correlated with the degree of insulin secreted. [53] One interesting study that administered intranasal insulin after meals found that insulin *increased* satiety and *decreased* food intake.[54]

If you're wondering why low-carb Paleo dieters frequently have higher satiety with less food, this is actually due primarily to higher protein intake—not anything to do with carbohydrates or insulin.[55] (We will discuss this more in upcoming sections.)

It is actually well known among nutrition scientists that insulin suppresses appetite.

The argument that carbs make you hungry is largely based on the previously discussed idea that those with insulin-producing tumors or who inject insulin frequently take in more food and become fatter. As we discussed, insulin in isolation—out of context of normal physiology—can produce increased food intake. But this is why good science doesn't operate with this sort of reductionism. For example, amylin—which is also secreted after ingesting carbohydrates—*suppresses* appetite. Based on this same reductionist logic of reducing everything down to one hormone (e.g., "carbs make you fat because

---

48 Taubes, G. Good Calories, Bad Calories

49 http://www.ncbi.nlm.nih.gov/pubmed/12499328

50 http://www.ncbi.nlm.nih.gov/pubmed/8862476

51 http://www.ncbi.nlm.nih.gov/pubmed/10435117

52 http://www.ncbi.nlm.nih.gov/pubmed/10567012

53 http://www.ncbi.nlm.nih.gov/pubmed/20456814

54 http://www.ncbi.nlm.nih.gov/pmc/articles/PMC3314365/

55 http://www.ncbi.nlm.nih.gov/pubmed/22935440

of the insulin"), we could say, "Carbs *suppress* appetite and cause fat loss because of the amylin." The same is true for leptin, which is also secreted much more strongly after eating carbs rather than fats.[56] Leptin boosts metabolism and suppresses appetite.[57] So based on the same sort of silly reductionist logic of looking at nutrition through the lens of a single hormone, we could say, "Carbohydrates suppress appetite and simultaneously boost your metabolism because of the leptin." And, in fact, real obesity scientists consider leptin—not insulin—to be the major hormone that regulates body fat levels. So if we were inclined try to myopically fixate on single macronutrients and to reduce everything down to one hormone that is critical for body fat regulation, we could actually make the argument that carbs help the body decrease body fat levels based on their effect on leptin. **But this isn't actually how body fat regulation happens! Body fat regulation happens in concert with dozens of different hormones operating in feedback with one another—not due to one individual hormone going up or down in response to a meal.** The point is that one can make all manner of silly arguments supporting basically *anything* so long as they operate with the sort of logic that tries to reduce everything down to one hormone. Physiology is complex, and this type of reductionist logic has no place in real scientific discussions.

Now, let's look at the effects of insulin on "calories out" (i.e., Taubes' notion that insulin causes laziness and lethargy). Again, fortunately for us, this theory has also been tested in several studies.

What did they find?

Several studies have found that higher fasting insulin is associated with a *higher* resting energy expenditure, independent of body fatness, not a lower expenditure. [58] [59] This is precisely the *opposite* of what Taubes' theory would predict. Other studies that have looked at the direct effects of spiking insulin on calorie expenditure have consistently shown that diets that vary in

---

56 http://www.ncbi.nlm.nih.gov/pubmed/10567012?dopt=AbstractPlus

57 http://www.ncbi.nlm.nih.gov/pubmed/9311966

58 http://www.ncbi.nlm.nih.gov/pubmed/10426380

59 http://www.ncbi.nlm.nih.gov/pubmed/16920075

carbohydrate to fat ratios do not create ***any*** measurable effects on calorie expenditure, even over long periods of time.[60] [61]

So if carbohydrates are not causing increased food intake or decreased calorie expenditure from lowered metabolic rate or laziness, then how exactly are they supposedly making us fat?

---

60 http://www.ncbi.nlm.nih.gov/pubmed/2058571

61 http://www.ncbi.nlm.nih.gov/pubmed/9497169

Carbs Turn into Body Fat? Hardly! But Dietary Fat Does So Rather Easily

One of the most glaring problems with the insulin-leads-to-fatness theory is this simple and obvious fact: **Dietary fat can also be stored as body fat—without any need for insulin spikes from carbohydrates.**

Did you imagine that with low-carb diets, somehow calories didn't matter anymore and you could eat all the fat you wanted without getting fat? I hope no one actually believes that.

But as it turns out, head low-carb guru Gary Taubes has essentially stated exactly that:

> **"You can't eat carbs, (but) you can basically exercise as much gluttony as you want as long you're eating fat and protein."**[62]

In order for Taubes to be correct—that is, in order for carbohydrates/insulin to be the major cause of fat gain—it would mean that carbohydrates would have to be converted to fatty acids and stored as body fat more efficiently than dietary fats can be stored. Or perhaps that somehow dietary fats cannot be stored as body fat—that maybe they are preferentially burned off as energy rather than stored as body fat. In order for Taubes' statement to have any truth, one of these two things must be going on.

Yet, there is a mountain of scientific research suggesting just the opposite—that the amount of calories you eat, not the amount of carbs or fat in your diet, or insulin in your body, is what dictates fat gain or fat loss. **Numerous studies have shown that high-carbohydrate and low-carbohydrate diets cause precisely equal amounts of fat loss or fat gain when matched for calories. In fact, virtually every metabolic ward study ever conducted in the history of nutritional**

---

62 (See HERE, starting from the 8 minute mark).

science has shown absolutely no difference in fat loss between low-carb and high-carb diets. [63] [64]

Moreover, despite the fact that low-carb advocates would have you believe that fat cannot be stored without insulin (and, by inference, carbohydrates), the fact is that dietary fat is readily stored with the help of the ASP (acylation stimulating protein). ASP may well play the major role in the uptake of fatty acids. By stimulating the enzyme that converts them to the triglyceride storage form, it is responsible for the fat cells "sucking up" fats from the bloodstream, while insulin is involved mainly in the *inhibition* of fat release from fat cells. So even without carbohydrate-induced insulin spikes, dietary fat can most definitely be stored as body fat. [65] [66] (Moreover, as mentioned previously, even if you avoid carbs completely but still eat some protein—which you will, since you can't live off dietary fat alone—you are *still* stimulating insulin from the protein to levels far exceeding those required to store fat and inhibit the release of fats from fat cells.) Thus, a low-carb diet does not really do anything to avoid fat storage—you still have the minimal amounts of insulin in the system to inhibit lipolysis, and even if you were to eat nothing but fat, you would still have ASP working to promote fat storage.

What's more, if the low-carbers were looking for a specific macronutrient that turns to body fat readily, dietary fat *is* stored as body fat much more easily and efficiently than carbohydrates are because there's no conversion needed at all. (However, this doesn't have any relevance to how fat or lean you are, because just as we have stated numerous times, it is calories—not the proportion of carbs or fat in the diet—that determines how fat or lean you are.)

But just for the sake of exploration, let's consider this notion that "carbs turn into fat."

---

63 Colpo, A. (2012, June 29). Finally, a study that proves a low-carb metabolic advantage? Yeah, Right… Retrieved from http://anthonycolpo.com/finally-a-study-that-proves-a-low-carb-metabolic-advantage-yeah-right/

64 Schoeller, D. A., & Buchholz, A. C. (2005). Energetics of obesity and weight control: Does diet composition matter? J Am Diet Assoc, 105(5 Suppl 1), S24-8.

65 http://carbsanity.blogspot.com/2012/06/fat-tissue-regulation-part-ix-asp-lpl.html

66 http://www.bodyrecomposition.com/fat-loss/insulin-levels-and-fat-loss-qa.html/

The process by which carbs "turn into fat" is called *de novo lipogenesis* (DNL), which is Latin for the "creation of new fat." And it is true—carbohydrates can indeed be turned into fat through DNL. The only problem is that virtually every study ever done on this subject has shown that the biochemical pathway of converting carbs to fat is so minute and inefficient that it contributes virtually nothing measurable to body fat.

- "Thus, de novo hepatic lipogenesis is a quantitatively minor pathway."[67]
- "DNL is not the pathway of first resort for added dietary CHO (carbohydrates) in humans, at least on Western (high-fat) diets. DNL can occur, but it generally does not. **A 'functional block' therefore exists between CHO and fat in humans, analogous to the absolute biochemical block in the direction from fat to carbohydrate in all animals."**[68]
- "Eucaloric replacement of dietary fat by CHO does not induce hepatic DNL to any substantial degree. Similarly, addition of CHO to a mixed diet does not increase hepatic DNL to quantitatively important levels, as long as CHO energy intake remains less than total energy expenditure (TEE)."[69]

The simple fact is that unless you're either eating absolutely massive amounts of carbohydrates (fulfilling over 100% of total daily calorie expenditure) for multiple days or eating an extreme low-fat diet, the human body simply does not convert carbohydrates to fat to any significant degree.

Remember, carbs cannot work to cause fat gain simply by keeping fat trapped in fat cells—that would only cause you to *maintain your current level of body fatness*. In order to actually *get fatter*, something—some kind of calories—has to be getting turned into fat and piled on top of existing amounts of body fat. And if carbs do not convert into fats, then where is that body fat coming from?

Well, primarily from dietary fat, of course.

When you actually do consume an excess of calories beyond the body's calorie expenditure, it is specifically the dietary fat you're

---

67 http://www.ncbi.nlm.nih.gov/pubmed/2022750

68 http://www.ncbi.nlm.nih.gov/pubmed/10365981

69 http://www.ncbi.nlm.nih.gov/pubmed/10365981

eating—not the carbohydrates—that actually gets turned into body fat.[70] It makes no logical sense that the body would go through the inefficient process of converting carbohydrates into fat to store them as body fat when it can just shunt dietary fat direct into body fat stores. And the science confirms that this is indeed the case--in a caloric excess, it's the dietary fat you're consuming that actually ends up in your body's fat cells, not the carbohydrates.

So if they were looking for a specific macronutrient to blame fat gain on, it's quite odd that they decided to get so creative in their efforts to blame carbohydrates when basic physiology shows us that fat is much more easily stored as body fat than carbohydrate is. The simple fact is that if you overconsume calories beyond your body's needs, the fats you eat in your diet will accumulate on your body as body fat regardless of how much carbohydrate you are (or aren't) eating.

So already here we see a fatal flaw in the argument: If carbs can only cause fat accumulation when eaten with fats, then how can one say it's *specifically* the carbs or *specifically* the fat that is "causing" the fat gain? If carbohydrates and insulin by themselves cannot even create body fat—and we still require dietary fat in order to actually store fat and accumulate more body fat—then is it the carbs or the fat that's making you fat? If you need *both,* then why demonize just one of them—why demonize carbohydrates when it's actually dietary fat that is the source of the fats that are stored in your fat cells?

To take this a step further, the notion that dietary fat only gets stored as body fat when carbohydrates are present is completely false. As we already saw with the discussion on ASP, dietary fat can be stored as body fat just fine without any insulin spike from carbohydrates. With or without carbohydrate-induced insulin spikes, dietary fat is mostly stored as body fat. [71]

Yes, eating 500 calories of carbohydrates will cause your fat to be "locked away" in fat cells instead of being burned off, but so will eating 500 calories of dietary fat.

This is a succinct breakdown of how the various macronutrients are stored and oxidized, as explained by Lyle McDonald:

---

70 http://wholehealthsource.blogspot.com/2011/08/carbohydrate-hypothesis-of-obesity.html

71 http://diabetes.diabetesjournals.org/content/56/1/168.full.pdf

1) Carbs are rarely converted to fat and stored as such.
2) When you eat more carbs, you burn more carbs and less fat; eat fewer carbs and you burn fewer carbs and more fat.
3) Protein is basically never going to be converted to fat and stored as such.
4) When you eat more protein, you burn more protein (and by extension, fewer carbs and less fat); eat less protein and you burn less protein (and by extension, more carbs and more fat).
5) Ingested dietary fat is primarily stored; eating more of it doesn't impact fat oxidation to a significant degree.[72]

A diet with any combination of macronutrients can make you fat (if there is an overall calorie excess). But the macronutrients do so through different mechanisms. To show you how this plays out, let's use the example of someone eating a diet that is 500 calories above the amount of calories they burn each day, but while on diets dominant in either carbs, protein, or fat:

MACRONUTRIENT (assume 500 calorie excess in each case)	MECHANISM	RESULT
CARBS	Excess dietary carbohydrate can make you fat (by impairing fat oxidation, such that more of your dietary fat intake ends up in your fat cells at the end of the day).	On a very high-carbohydrate diet, 500 calories worth of dietary fat will end up being stored in your fat cells instead of burned off, at the end of the day.
PROTEIN	Excess dietary protein can make you fat (by impairing fat oxidation, such that more of your dietary fat intake ends up in your fat cells at the end of the day).	On a very high-protein diet, 500 calories worth of dietary fat will end up being stored in your fat cells instead of burned off, at the end of the day.
FAT	Excess dietary fat can make you fat by being directly stored in fat cells.	On a very high-fat diet, 500 calories worth of dietary fat will end up being stored in your fat cells instead of burned off, at the end of the day.

72 http://www.bodyrecomposition.com/fat-loss/how-we-get-fat.html/

And we already know this is true because *we have done the studies!* When people are overfed on diets rich in either carbs or fat, **"[and] the same number of calories are overfed, the same amount of fat is gained."**[73] [74]

In other words, if there is an overall caloric excess, eating a diet dominant in *any macronutrient* causes your fat to be "locked away" in your fat cells instead of being burned off.

Yet somehow, all of these basic facts of physiology have been ignored by low-carb diet advocates who have promoted this pseudoscientific narrative about how carbs/sugars are uniquely fattening. It's just wrong—plain and simple.

First of all, if you are eating an amount of calories at or below how many calories you burn each day, then *precisely none* of the food you are eating—whether your diet is 90% carbohydrates or 90% fat—will accumulate as body fat. If you *are* taking in more calories than you burn, both carbs and fat can be turned into body fat—so you can get fat on a zero-carb diet of nothing but meat and cream, or a fruitarian diet where 99% of your calories are sugars. Now, if you have a caloric excess while eating a mixed diet of both some fats and some carbohydrates (as virtually every normal person is doing), it is preferentially dietary fat—not carbs—that becomes fat on your body. And again, you do *not* have to be eating a carb-rich diet for dietary fat to be stored as body fat.

The point here is simply this: You can take in all the insulin-boosting carbs you want, but as long as you are eating at or below your maintenance level of calories, you will not gain an ounce of fat. Similarly, you can eat a zero-carb diet where 90% of your calories are from fats and avoid insulin "spikes" completely, and if you eat *more* calories than your body requires, you'll still get fat.

---

73 http://www.bodyrecomposition.com/fat-loss/is-a-calorie-a-calorie.html/

74 http://www.ncbi.nlm.nih.gov/pubmed/7598063

The Real Test: What Happens When You Put Overweight People on Low-Carb Diets vs. Higher-Carb Diets?

If carbohydrates/insulin—rather than calories—were the key factor in fat gain and fat loss, then at equal calories, a low-carb diet should cause more fat loss than a high-carb diet. For example, a 1,500-calorie diet that is low in carbs should cause more fat loss than a 1,500-calorie diet that is high in carbs.

This has been tested in numerous studies and found to be false.

The research has proven over and over again that when low-carb diets are compared to higher-carb diets of equal calories, low-carb diets offer no benefits whatsoever—for either health or fat loss. Nada. Zilch.

This was the conclusion from the latest 2014 meta-analysis (i.e., data from a non-cherry-picked comprehensive review of the scientific studies) on the subject: **"There is probably little or no difference in weight loss and changes in cardiovascular risk factors up to two years of follow-up when overweight and obese adults, with or without type 2 diabetes, are randomized to low CHO (low-carb) diets and isoenergetic balance (higher-carb diets that are equal in calories)."** [75]

In other words, looking at all these different studies that compared people on equal calorie low-carb and higher-carb diets, they were not able to detect *any difference whatsoever* in either health measures or fat loss.

So is this meta-analysis telling us something novel? Not really. As it turns out, there are dozens of studies that have found this conclusion, going back several decades.

Numerous studies have compared low-carb diets to higher-carb diets. In metabolic ward studies (Grey and Kipnis, [76] Golay et al.,[77]

---

75 (http://www.plosone.org/article/info%3Adoi%2F10.1371%2Fjournal.pone.0100652)

76 http://www.maxcondition.com/page.php?152

77 Golay A, et al. (1996). Similar weight loss with low or high carbohydrate diets. Am J Clin Nutr. 63:174-8.

Miyashita et al.,[78] Stimnson et al.,[79] and Naude et al.[80]), **researchers consistently find no difference in fat loss between those on low-carb and high-carb diets.**

Even when we compare higher-carb diets to *extremely* low-carbohydrate diets, we see the same thing: as long as protein intake and calories are controlled, **there is no difference in fat loss between high- and low-carb diets.**

- A relatively recent trial examined the effects of three diets consisting of roughly 1400 kcals each day for twelve weeks. The diets had the following macronutrient proportions: a) very low fat and high carb (70% carb), b) moderate carb (50% carb), and c) very low carb (4% carb). What did they find? There were no differences in fat loss between the groups. [81]
- Another recent trial compared two 1500-calorie diets, a moderate carbohydrate diet (40% carbohydrate) and a very low-carb ketogenic diet (a tiny 5% carbohydrate). The researchers concluded that the "diets were equally effective in reducing body weight and insulin resistance, but the ketogenic low-carb diet was associated with several adverse metabolic and emotional effects."[82] In other words, going low carb did not accomplish any additional fat loss—all it did was make people feel worse.
- Grey and Kipnis (1971) studied ten obese patients who were fed 1,500 liquid-formula diets containing either 72% or 0% carbohydrate for four weeks before switching to the other diet. **Despite massive differences in insulin levels, participants lost the same amount of weight each week regardless of**

78 http://anthonycolpo.com/finally-a-study-that-proves-a-low-carb-metabolic-advantage-yeah-right/

79 http://www.ncbi.nlm.nih.gov/pubmed/17785367

80 http://www.plosone.org/article/info%3Adoi%2F10.1371%2Fjournal.pone.0100652

81 (http://www.ncbi.nlm.nih.gov/pubmed/16403234)

82 (http://www.ncbi.nlm.nih.gov/pubmed/16685046)

> **whether they ate the high-carbohydrate diet or the zero-carbohydrate diet.** [83]

These studies make it abundantly clear that there is simply no validity to the claims that carbohydrates or insulin have some thermodynamics-transcending fattening effect.

In calorie-controlled experiments where they put groups of people on equal calorie diets that are either high-carb/low-fat or low-carb/high-fat, studies consistently show that weight goes up or down by the same amounts at a given level of calories.

Some studies have been conducted where participants are put on deliberately fattening diets (i.e., overfeeding calories), where one diet is low in carbohydrates and high in fats, and the other diet is high in carbohydrates. The diets are equal in total calories. What do these studies show?

The first one by Lammert et al. took ten pairs of lean young men and overfed them by 1,195 kcal per day for 21 days. One group was given the carbohydrate-rich diet and the other a fat-rich diet. Subjects lived and ate in a research setting the entire time, so calories taken in and burned were controlled for extremely well. The researchers analyzed body composition weekly by underwater weighing. What did they find? Both groups gained very similar amounts of total weight, and the increase in body fat mass was virtually identical.[84] Another similar study by Horton et al. reached the same conclusion. In fact, in Horton's study, they found that carbohydrate overfeeding caused only 75-85% of excess calories to be stored as body fat, while with fat overfeeding, 90-95% of excess calories were stored as fat.[85] They concluded, **"Excess dietary fat leads to greater fat accumulation than does excess dietary carbohydrate, and the difference was greatest early in the overfeeding period."**[86] So, if anything, the research indicates that fat calories are more easily stored as body fat than carbohydrates.

Under non-overfeeding conditions—that is, where participants are given an amount of calories that will cause them to maintain their

---

83 http://www.nejm.org/doi/full/10.1056/NEJM197110072851504

84 http://169.229.201.201/hellerstein-lab/pdfs/grunnet.pdf

85 http://www.ncbi.nlm.nih.gov/pubmed/7598063

86 http://www.ncbi.nlm.nih.gov/pubmed/7598063

normal body weight—the results are very similar. Renowned obesity researchers Rudolph Leibel, MD, and Jules Hirsch, MD, did a fantastic experiment where participants were kept under metabolic ward conditions for not just weeks, but months. They gave the participants a diet of either high carbohydrates or high fat for many months, and then after that, switched the same people to an equal calorie diet with the opposite macronutrient profile—so if they were eating low carb/high fat before, they would now be eating a high-carb/low-fat diet, and vice versa. Here's a summary of their findings:

> "We showed that the carbohydrate-to-fat ratio could vary widely with little or no alteration in the energy requirement for weight maintenance. The results of a 13-week study in which an individual was fed a formula diet extremely rich in carbohydrate and low in fat for a period of 38 (days) [were that] weight varied little throughout the study and average energy intake was the same throughout... **The reason for emphasizing these findings is that, under the strict conditions imposed by hospitalization and feedings of a formula diet, energy needs are the same over long periods of time even though carbohydrate-to-fat ratios vary.**"[87] [88]

In other words, when calories are the same, you can vary carbohydrate and fat intakes massively with absolutely no differences in body weight.

We have the science on the subject. We don't need to guess or speculate. This subject is not still open for debate or waiting for more studies to be conducted. We have done the studies already.

Virtually every metabolic ward study that has been conducted on the subject for the last 75 years has repeatedly shown that

87 http://wholehealthsource.blogspot.com

88 http://www.ncbi.nlm.nih.gov/pubmed/1734671

when calories are equal, there is no difference in fat loss between low-carb and high-carb diets. [89] [90] [91] [92] [93] [94]

A comprehensive review of studies found that there is no metabolic advantage for low-carb diets. [95]

If the low-carb gurus are right and carbohydrate restriction creates some state of magical fat-loss physiology that goes beyond the number of calories that are restricted, then why is this effect virtually never detected in controlled scientific studies?

To put this more plainly, we can safely say that there is no magical thermodynamic transcending effect of low-carb diets, or that if there is an effect, it is so small as to be utterly meaningless.

Low-carb diets make you lean only to the extent that you eat fewer overall calories. And in such a scenario, a higher-carbohydrate diet of equal calories will work just as well.

---

89 http://www.ncbi.nlm.nih.gov/pubmed/15867892

90 http://ajcn.nutrition.org/content/68/6/1157.full.pdf,

91 http://www.ncbi.nlm.nih.gov/pubmed/8363199

92 http://www.ncbi.nlm.nih.gov/pubmed/11374180

93 http://ajcn.nutrition.org/content/63/2/174.abstract

94 http://www.ncbi.nlm.nih.gov/pubmed/2319073)

95 http://www.ncbi.nlm.nih.gov/pubmed/15867892

Why Do Some People Lose Weight Eating Low-Carb?

Even though we have shown you through numerous studies that carbohydrates and insulin are not linked to body fatness in any significant way, there is still one glaring reality to account for: the many thousands of people who have lost weight by following low-carb diets.

This, according to the low-carb gurus, is "proof" that low-carb works. "So what if the studies often contradict our ideas about carbohydrates and insulin? The simple fact is that low-carb works to cause people to lose weight, so therefore our theories are right even if the metabolic ward studies don't show it—it is still carbohydrates and insulin that are the problem even though the studies don't prove us right."

So what could possibly account for these people's weight-loss results on low-carb diets? If people do frequently lose weight on low-carb diets, then why bother with all this theory and all these studies—people lose weight, so carbohydrate avoidance must work, right?

If what we have explained so far in this book is true, then you're probably wondering how it's possible that many studies have shown weight loss on low-carbohydrate, higher-fat diets.

There is, after all, quite a bit of good scientific evidence to support the notion that low-carb diets are effective for weight loss. That is an unquestionable and non-debatable fact. The part that is highly questionable and debatable is whether that weight loss has anything whatsoever to do with carbohydrates and insulin.

The truth is that the reason so-called "low-carb" diets frequently cause fat loss is *not* actually due to the carbohydrate restriction itself!

There are three major reasons why so-called "low-carb diets" cause weight loss that can entirely account for the observed phenomenon that these diets often do result in people losing weight (and none of them have to do with insulin or the inherent metabolic effects of carbohydrates):

1) **Removal of major food groups reduces overall calorie intake.** Any time you ask someone to remove a large portion of their normal diet—whether carbs (as in low-carb diets), fat (as in low-fat diets), or animal foods (as in veganism)—*overall calorie intake drops significantly*. Thus, there is an enormous difference between *adding fats* into a diet to make the diet a high-

fat diet versus *removing carbohydrates*. You can arrive at a relatively lower-carb, higher-fat diet by either method, but only the latter—removal of carbohydrates—will drive overall calories down and create fat loss. The former—adding fats into the diet—will tend to create fat *gain*. This effect of lowering total calorie intake by removing a major food group is also seen with both low-fat diets and vegan diets, which also are scientifically proven to cause fat loss and improve health markers. The simple fact is that any diet that asks you to reduce/eliminate one entire macronutrient like carbs (low-carb diets) or fats (low-fat diets) will cause fat loss. This isn't because carbs are uniquely fattening or that fats are uniquely fattening, and thus removing them causes this amazing fat loss that transcends the laws of thermodynamics. It's that any dietary intervention that removes a major food group tends to lower overall calories consumed—simply by virtue of removing a source of calories, and also likely by lowering the food reward/palatability factor in the diet, and thus, the intervention causes fat loss. (Note: Food reward/palatability will be discussed extensively in the next chapter.) Anyone who tries to explain this effect via the inherent metabolic properties of carbs or fats (e.g., "eating low-carb makes you lean because it lowers insulin levels") is preaching inaccurate pseudoscience. Removing *any macronutrient* from the diet will cause fat loss due to changes in overall calories consumed—and the weight loss that is achieved is in precise relationship to the decrease in the amount of calories consumed.

2) **Shifting from processed foods to whole foods lowers overall calorie intake.** In addition to removing major food groups that comprise a large portion of people's diets, most low-carb Paleo diets emphasize getting rid of processed foods and shifting to whole foods. For anyone who is eating a processed food diet, this shift has a dramatic effect on lowering the reward value of the diet and, by virtue of that, will lower overall calorie intake even more. In many cases, this simple strategy alone will cause large amounts of fat loss.[96]

---

96 http://wholehealthsource.blogspot.com/2009/09/paleolithic-diet-clinical-trials-part.html

3) **Protein! Higher protein consumption lowers overall calorie intake.** This is the biggest one. Most so-called "low-carb" diets don't actually drive fat loss due to carbohydrate restriction. They do it primarily due to *increased protein consumption*! Low-carb diets often emphasize lots of protein and meat consumption. This is proven to very powerfully increase satiety, lower food reward, and drive down overall calories consumed by hundreds of calories per day in some cases. [97] [98] [99]

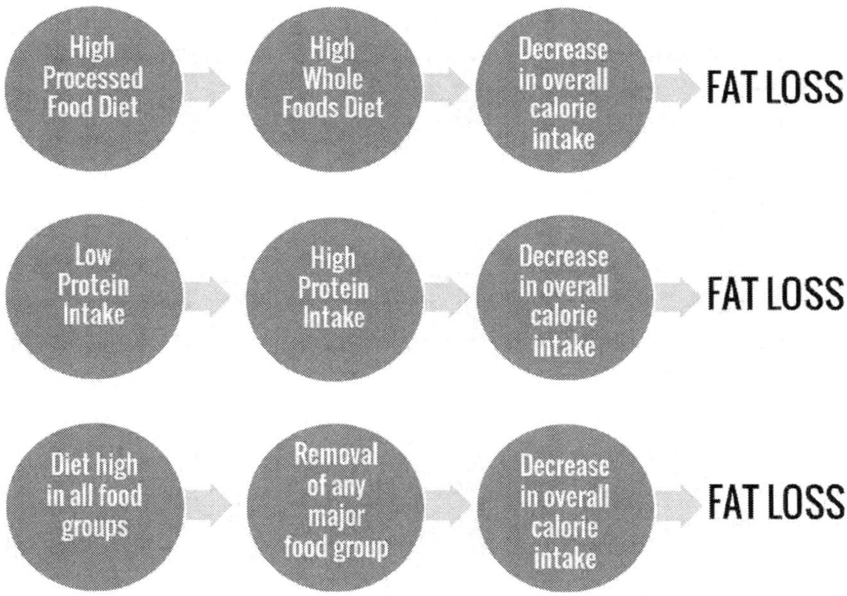

The reason low-carb diets work for weight loss—when they actually do work—is *not* due to the metabolic effects of carbohydrates themselves or anything to do with insulin. Rather, it is the simple result of decreasing overall *calorie* intake. To the extent that a "low-carb" diet causes you to reduce your overall calorie intake, it will cause fat loss. To the extent that you eat a low-

97 http://www.ncbi.nlm.nih.gov/pubmed/16002798

98 http://carbsanity.blogspot.com/2010/04/high-protein-diet-induces-sustained.html

99 http://www.ncbi.nlm.nih.gov/pubmed/15867892

carbohydrate diet *without* reducing your calorie intake, you will *not* lose weight. (There are, in fact, some notable low-carb gurus who are still extremely overweight and have even gained weight in recent years, despite eating extreme low-carb diets for years.)

The point is that neither the amount of carbohydrates nor the amount of fats you're eating is a significant factor in fat loss. This is why we can see lean people on very high-carbohydrate diets or very high-fat diets—neither is incompatible with being lean. The real factors responsible for fat loss are removal of major food groups a person eats, shifting from processed foods to whole foods, and increasing protein consumption. (Even more than that, the effect has to do with palatability and food reward—factors that will be explained in the next chapter.)

These are the three *secret* factors responsible for the weight loss of "low-carb" diets. It has nothing to do with lowering insulin levels or any other such metabolic effects of carbohydrate restriction. The same exact weight loss effect (and health benefits) can be achieved on a diet high in carbohydrates that emphasizes removal of fatty foods from the diet, shifts a person away from processed foods towards fruits and vegetables, and has a high protein intake. And this is confirmed by an important recent study comparing the weight loss effects of different popular diets that vary dramatically in macronutrient ratios, which find that after a long period of time, **weight loss is roughly the same regardless of which of these diets you go on.**[100]

The idea that the carbohydrates consumed are a major factor in fat gain and fat loss is simply false—it is a distraction from the real factors at play.

Basically, what's really going on here is this: the advocates of these diets are essentially just using their diet rules to trick you into unknowingly lowering your caloric intake while simultaneously telling you "calories don't matter" and convincing you that this effect is due to something about the inherent metabolic or hormonal effects of carbohydrates.

We already know that this is wrong.

Yet, as of recent years, there are numerous studies (which have been highly publicized in the media) that appear to show that when "low-carb diets" are compared to "low-fat diets," low-carb diets achieve

---

100 http://www.ncbi.nlm.nih.gov/pubmed/25182101

greater fat loss. In fact, the latest of these studies[101] was just published prior to this writing (in Sept. 2014) and has garnered much press in mainstream media outlets with bold proclamations of "Low carb beats low fat for weight loss."

The problem with this study is that, in reality, it didn't compare low-carb dieters to low-fat dieters at all! The low-carb participants were asked to restrict their baseline levels of carbohydrate intake by a whopping 75%—from 240 grams per day all the way down to a paltry 40 grams of digestible carbohydrate per day while the so-called "low-fat" participants were asked only to restrict their fat intake by 5% from their normal fat intake. 75% restriction of carbs from baseline compared to a measly 5% restriction of fat from their normal fat intake. Does this sound like a valid study to you? To put this another way, they allowed the "low-fat" group to take in up to 600 calories per day from fat, while they allowed the low-carb group to take in only 160 calories per day from carbohydrates. This experiment was not a study of "low carb vs. low fat" as was claimed. As Katz notes in his incisive analysis,[102] **it was really a study comparing one group that was put on a highly modified and heavily restricted diet to one that was hardly changed at all from their normal diet.** What a shock—the heavily restricted dieters lost more weight than the ones who didn't change their diet much.

Importantly, the study claimed that both groups took in a "similar" number of calories, but the low-carb dieters lost more fat (eight more pounds) over the course of the year. Thus, the researchers implied that low-carb dieters had a metabolic advantage in that they lost more fat despite eating essentially the same amount of calories. So maybe there is some magic to low-carb diets after all? Nope. If you actually look at the calorie intakes, the calorie intakes were not so "similar." The low-carb group took in an average of 79 calories fewer per day than the "low fat" group.

So was the weight loss due to eating low carb or simply eating fewer calories?

Let's do some basic math and find out. 79 calories less per day for a year (365 days) = nearly 29,000 fewer calories. There are roughly 3,500 calories in a pound of fat. So 29,000 divided by 3,500 = just over

---

101 http://annals.org/article.aspx?articleid=1900694

102 http://www.huffingtonpost.com/david-katz-md/post_8304_b_5752160.html

8. That just so happens to be the exact amount of additional pounds that the low-carb group lost compared to the other group. **The weight loss was entirely accounted for by the lower calorie intake. If the so-called "low-fat" group had lowered their calorie intake to the same extent, they would've lost the same exact amount of weight.**

In all of the studies that appear to show that low-carb diets provided superior weight loss, they almost universally fail to control for calorie intake. When low carb proves to be comparatively superior for weight loss to other diets, it's typically due to slight differences in overall calories consumed. In studies that *do* control for calorie intake, there is virtually never an advantage for low-carb diets.

Another massive confounding variable that contaminates the results of the majority of studies purporting to compare "low-carb" to "low-fat" diets is the absence of controlling for protein intake. Higher protein intake is a very reliable way to cause a person to spontaneously and unconsciously lower their *overall calorie intake.* Most of these so-called "low-carb" diets are also higher protein diets, thus they frequently decrease overall calorie intake more than the "low-fat" (and lower protein) diet, and yet, we frequently see silly headlines based on such fatally flawed studies claiming, "Low carb beats low fat." **If those on a low-carb diet lost more weight, it is because they restricted calories more, which is an effect largely driven by the higher protein intake, not because of the inherent metabolic effects of eating fewer carbohydrates.**[103]

The studies that have claimed to show some weight loss advantage for low-carb diets invariably fail to control for protein intake. So what they're really doing is *not* comparing a low-carb diet to a high-carb diet—they're comparing a low-carb, *high-protein* diet to a higher carbohydrate, *lower protein* diet. This is not a valid comparison, since higher protein intake will reliably lead to more fat loss regardless of the carbohydrate or fat content of the diet.

What happens when studies control for protein intake—like, for example, administering diets that are either high-carb or low-carb but otherwise matched for protein and calories? Studies invariably find that

---

103 103 http://www.ncbi.nlm.nih.gov/pubmed/15867892

the fat loss does not depend on the carbohydrate restriction and is solely due to the effect of protein.[104]

When calorie and protein intake are controlled for, the apparent weight-loss advantage that some studies appear to show for low-carb diets magically disappears.

As sports nutritionist Alan Aragon states:

> "A key point that must be made is that the research is not sufficient grounds to be dogmatic about low-carbing in the first place. On the whole, studies do not match protein intakes between diets. Adequate protein intakes have multiple advantages (i.e., LBM [lean body mass] support, satiety, thermic effect), and they simply end up being compared to inadequate protein intakes. Thus, it's not lower carb intake per se that imparts any advantage, it's the higher protein intake. Once you match protein intake between diets, the one with more carbs is actually the one with the potential for a slight metabolic advantage. Furthermore, the majority of the research compares dietary extremes (high-carb/low-fat/low-protein versus low-carb/high-fat/moderate-protein). **The funny part is, the majority of long-term trials (twelve months or more) *still* fail to show a significant weight loss difference.** Note that these trials use the sedentary obese, so in the fit population, any weight loss differences would be even more miniscule."[105]

But perhaps the biggest confounding variable of all in these studies that purport to be comparing "low-carb" and "low-fat" diets—and a factor that is almost universally not considered by lay people and even the researchers themselves—is food reward and overall palatability of these diets. We will go into depth on food reward/palatability in the next chapter, but suffice it to say that the palatability (overall pleasure and pleasantness of taste one derives from the diet) is **largely determined by the specific food choices one makes, not the overall macronutrient content of the diet.**

In simple terms, depending on the specific food choices one makes, you can end up with either a highly palatable and extremely gourmet and delicious high-carb, low-fat diet, or a very low palatability high-

104 http://www.ncbi.nlm.nih.gov/pubmed/22935440

105 http://www.maxcondition.com/page.php?152

carb, low-fat diet. Similarly, you can end up with a very high palatability low-carb, high-fat diet or a very low palatability low-carb, high-fat diet. Many of these studies that attempt to compare "low-carb" to "low-fat" diets completely ignore considerations of reward and palatability and how they affect overall calories consumed. Thus, many times these researchers ascribe differences they see between these diets to the inherent metabolic effects of either carbohydrates or fats, when really all that's going on is that the group that was given the tastier and more pleasurable diet simply ate more total calories. There are studies that point to this fact as well—since on diets where people are allowed to eat however much they want, sometimes low-fat diets cause more weight loss than low-carb diets and sometimes low-carb diets cause more weight loss than low-fat diets, while when precisely matched for calories, they cause equal weight loss. Therefore, these differences are likely NOT pointing to differences in the effects of carbs or fats, but the fact that one diet is more pleasurable and stimulates more overall calorie consumption. There is even one recent study that compared a traditional Western diet (34% fat, 16% protein, 50% carbohydrate) to a traditional Asian diet (15% fat, 15% protein, 70% carbohydrate), where even though researchers made attempts to have each group eat the same number of calories, people lost weight on the high-carb, low-fat diet and gained weight on the higher fat, lower carb diet. [106]

Again, this is likely NOT due to the inherent metabolic effects of either fats or carbohydrates but due to the effects of palatability of the diet influencing overall calories consumed.

We can't emphasize just how enormous of a confounding factor reward/palatability is, and how universally it is failed to be considered by people involved in the fat versus carb macronutrient wars. Wherever a study shows that one diet outperformed another in terms of weight loss (i.e., where a "low-carb" diet outperforms a "low-fat" diet), it's extremely likely that this effect is *not* due to the inherent metabolic effects of fat or carbohydrates, but rather is due to slight differences in the *palatability* of the specific foods consumed in those diets. Yet there are countless "gurus" out there who routinely interpret the findings of such studies as evidence of the effects of macronutrients (carbohydrates and fat). **To put this very directly: the**

106 http://wholehealthsource.blogspot.com/2014/10/metabolic-effects-of-traditional-asian.html

vast majority of studies examining ad libitum (eating as much as one desires) diets that purport to compare "low-carb" to "low-fat" diets are largely *invalid* due to failing to control for overall palatability of the diet.

When discussing whether low-carb or low-fat diets are better for fat loss, it is worth reemphasizing that we already know this from dozens of metabolic ward studies—when low-carb and high-carb diets of equal calories are compared, they provide the same exact amount of weight loss.[107] Remember, this *proves* that it is indeed calories—*not* carbohydrates/insulin—that dictate fat gain and fat loss.

Moreover, even in non-calorie-controlled studies, despite not controlling for protein intake or palatability of the diet, long-term differences between different diets are typically small. A brand new study (Sept 2014) compared the most popular diets around—everything from low-carb, high-fat Atkins diets to ultra-high-carb, low-fat vegan diets and everything in between from the Zone diet to the South Beach diet, and anything else you can think of. What did they find?

> **"Significant weight loss was observed with any low-carbohydrate or low-fat diet. Weight loss differences between individual named diets were small."[108]**

The truth is that despite all the constant hype around carbs and fats we've been bombarded with from the diet gurus over the last several decades, the science shows that diets that vary wildly in carbohydrate and fat content simply don't produce dramatically different results. As has been found in countless studies and numerous comprehensive literature reviews—the top of the hierarchy of scientific evidence—fat loss is dictated by overall calorie balance, not the inherent metabolic effects of carbohydrates or fats.

- **"In a 4-year prospective study, weight gain was not significantly influenced by dietary composition but rather by total energy intake."[109]**

---

107 http://www.ncbi.nlm.nih.gov/pubmed/19692216

108 http://www.ncbi.nlm.nih.gov/pubmed/25182101

109 http://ajcn.nutrition.org/content/78/4/834S.full

- This study reviewed the literature on the weight loss effectiveness of the most popular diets and concluded: **"Review of the literature suggests that weight loss is independent of diet composition. Energy restriction is the key variable associated with weight reduction in the short term."**[110]
- One of the few long-term studies comparing low-carb and low-fat diets concluded: **"There were no differences in weight, body composition, or bone mineral density between the groups at any time point."**[111]
- **Evidence abounds that low-carbohydrate diets present no significant advantage over more traditional energy-restricted, nutritionally balanced diets both in terms of weight loss and weight maintenance."**[112]

As researcher George Bray, MD, states very plainly and directly, **"Weight loss is related to adherence to the diet, not to its macronutrient composition."**[113]

None of this is to say that low-carb diets "don't work" or are "bad" or are less effective than many other types of diets that differ greatly in macronutrient composition. Most research indicates that they are about as effective as any other diet of equal calories.[114]

What this is saying is that all of the notions and theories promoted by low-carb gurus about carbs causing fat gain and low-carb diets causing some magical hormonal state that is conducive to fat loss are simply wrong. Some studies indicate that low-carb diets can be very slightly better than other diets in some cases, and very slightly worse in other cases. But apart from individual cherry-picked studies that may show low-carb diets to be either slightly better or slightly worse than some other diet, the literature reviews and meta-analyses on the subject

---

110 http://www.ncbi.nlm.nih.gov/pubmed/11320946

111 http://www.ncbi.nlm.nih.gov/pmc/articles/PMC2949959/

112 http://www.ncbi.nlm.nih.gov/pubmed/14672862

113 http://www.proteinpower.com/drmike/wp-content/uploads/2008/07/bray-review-of-gcbc.pdf

114 http://www.plosone.org/article/info%3Adoi%2F10.1371%2Fjournal.pone.0100652

are clear that low-carb diets are generally no better than other diets of equal calories.

For those inclined to the thinking, "But I lost 70 pounds on a low-carb diet, therefore the low-carb gurus must be right—carbs were making me fat, and I lost fat because of the lower insulin levels," consider this:

- Thousands of people have also lost huge amounts of weight on low-fat, high-carb diets.
- Thousands of people have lost huge amounts of weight on ultra-high-carb vegan or even fruitarian diets while consuming huge amounts of sugar.
- Thousands of people have lost huge amounts of weight while eating a nearly pure Rice Diet, and this was even a famous and very successful weight loss program at Duke University for decades.[115]
- Thousands of people have lost huge amounts of weight on the Potato Diet, which consists of eating nothing but high-glycemic, carbohydrate-filled potatoes all day, including, by the way, countless low-carb Paleo followers who have adopted the Potato Diet as a way to lose fat after their efforts stall on the low-carb diet.

So if you're trying to explain the weight loss that happens for some people on low-carb diets as an effect that is specifically *unique to eating a low-carb, high-fat diet,* do you think the above people should also explain their weight loss as a result of the inherent metabolic effects of eating carbohydrate-based diets, or the magic power of eating nothing but rice or potatoes?

There must be a more parsimonious explanation for fat loss that can account for the simple fact that countless people have lost fat successfully on diets of diametrically opposed macronutrient compositions.

And there is! According to Guyenet, "The best available evidence continues to suggest that the calorie value of food impacts body fatness, but macronutrient composition doesn't. I believe we'll eventually learn that the story is a bit more complex than that, but the

---

115 https://www.drmcdougall.com/misc/2013nl/dec/131200.pdf

boring adage 'a calorie is a calorie' is the interpretation the evidence currently supports."[116]

Consider this: if carbs/insulin were the main cause of fat gain, then the trend in comparison studies looking at low-carb versus low-fat diets would be that the very high-carb diets are not just less effective than low-carb diets for fat loss, but we would see that *only* those on low-carb diets lose fat, and those on the high-carb diets would actually *gain* fat. Yet, virtually all studies show that when matched for calories, they cause equal amounts of fat loss.

In non-calorie-matched studies, where one type of diet appears superior for fat loss over another diet—whether it's low-fat diets besting low-carb diets or low-carb diets besting low-fat diets—the effect likely has nothing to do with the carbohydrate to fat ratio of the diet and everything to do with how many total calories were consumed.

If carbohydrates and insulin were a major factor regulating body fat mass, this would be an incredibly easy thing to demonstrate. Yet, virtually every study that controls for calories and/or protein (i.e., every well-controlled study that is actually designed to look at the effects of carbohydrate) shows no such effect.

To support their case, low-carb advocates can only resort to cherry-picking poorly controlled studies that fail to control for either calories and/or protein. Why? **Because there is no body of calorie- and protein-controlled studies showing low-carb diets are superior.** As soon as well-controlled studies are conducted that allow us to directly assess the effects of carbohydrates/insulin, the "magic" of low-carb diets all of the sudden disappears.

If there is any fat loss advantage to eating low-carb at all, it is so utterly miniscule as to be completely undetectable by dozens of studies that have deliberately gone looking for it.

---

116 http://wholehealthsource.blogspot.com/2014/10/metabolic-effects-of-traditional-asian.html

Are Populations that Eat High-Carbohydrate Diets More Obese?

If we want to test out this theory that carbs and insulin cause fatness, one simple way of examining whether it is true is to find some cultures around the world that eat very high-carbohydrate diets and see how fat they are. It really is that simple, and this is not a theory that's difficult to test. If carbs cause you to be fat, any population group that consumes a lot of carbohydrates each day should have higher rates of overweight and obesity.

So let's have a look at some populations known for eating large amounts of carbohydrates and see if that's the case:

The Tukisenta tribe in New Guinea: According to Trowell and Burkitt in their book *Western Diseases,* the Tukisenta ate a diet consisting mostly of sweet potatoes, which was a whopping 94% carbohydrate. The men ate about 2,300 calories each day, and the women ate about 1,770 calories each day. The scientists who went to study this tribe found them to be fit, lean, and muscular. [117]

The population of the West Nile district in Uganda during the 1940s: The diet of this population consisted almost entirely of foods extremely rich in carbohydrates: cassava, bananas, millet, corn, lentils, peanuts, and vegetables. According to Trowell and Burkitt, despite a constant abundance of food, "in the 1940s it was quite unusual to see a stout man or woman." Trowell and Burkitt also noted that the only overweight people in the area were affluent people who deviated from the traditional starch-based diet.[118] This same trend has been noted in countless societies in Africa.

Nearly the entire continent of Asia during the 20th century: China, India, Japan, Taiwan, and many other countries in Asia eat traditional diets extremely high in carbohydrates. They are largely based on white rice, as well as root vegetables along with some fruit. Yet, up until the Westernization of these countries and incorporation of processed foods into their diet, overweight and obesity were nearly

117 http://wholehealthsource.blogspot.com/2010/11/glucose-tolerance-in-non-industrial.html

118 http://wholehealthsource.blogspot.com/2011/08/carbohydrate-hypothesis-of-obesity.html

unheard of in these populations. Traditional Chinese, Japanese, and Southern Indians were among the leanest people on the planet.[119]

The Pima Indians: The Pima Indians are a famous group within the obesity research community, largely because obesity rates are so incredibly high. But there's also something else interesting about this group—only about half of the Pima Indian population has a tendency to become obese. You see, as the United States defined its borders, the Pima Indian population—which was on the border of New Mexico in the United States and Mexico—got divided. Subsequently, after a drought of the Gila River, the US Pima Indians suffered famine and were rescued by government rations, which consisted of various processed foods and things like canned meats, white flour, vegetable oils, sugar, hydrogenated lard, and other canned foods. They subsequently became obese and have remained that way ever since. However, the Pima Indians on the Mexican side of the border that have largely remained on their traditional diet—which is lower in fat and significantly *higher* in starchy carbohydrates—have dramatically lower rates of diabetes and obesity. So let me summarize. These two population groups share the same genetics. The US Pima Indians have the highest obesity rates in the world (about 70%) while the Mexican Pima Indians have under 10%. Same genetics, but totally different rates of obesity. The Spanish were the group who first made contact with the Pima Indians back in 1539, and like all groups around the world on their traditional diet, the Spanish found them to be extremely lean and healthy. The traditional Pima diet was a high-carbohydrate diet consisting of beans, corn, and squash, with wild fish, game meat, and plants. *"Researchers at the NIDDK in Phoenix have estimated that the traditional Pima diet took about 70 percent of its calories in the form of carbohydrates, 15 percent in protein, and 15 percent in fat. By the 1950s, the proportions had changed to 61 percent carbohydrate, 15 percent in protein, and 24 percent in fat. In 1971 it was 44 percent carbohydrate, 12 percent protein, and 44 percent fat – a tripling of the fat content."*[120] During the span of time where they became the most obese population on Earth, carbohydrate content decreased dramatically and fat content of their diet tripled—clearly demonstrating that carbohydrates are not the source of obesity.

---

119 http://wholehealthsource.blogspot.com/2011/08/carbohydrate-hypothesis-of-obesity.html

120 Campos, P. The Obesity Myth.

The Pima Indians do not in any way show us that "carbohydrates make you fat." They show us that a diet based on processed foods makes you fat.

Kitava: Up until very recently—the 1990s—the people of the South Pacific island of Kitava had not been influenced by the Western diet and had continued eating the traditional diet that they'd eaten for centuries. Dr. Staffan Lindeberg researched this population heavily during the 1990s and found that their diet consisted mostly of taro, sweet potatoes, cassava, fruit, coconut, and seafood. They ate about 50g a day of unrefined sugar from fruit. Their diet came in at a whopping 69% carbohydrate. Lindeberg found that there were literally no cases of overweight or obesity on the entire island! The lone individual who was slightly overweight had left the island for several years to go live in the city. You may also be interested to know that their fasting insulin level (a measure of insulin resistance and diabetes) was extremely low, and that diabetes and heart disease were unheard of on the island. A diet that is 69% carbohydrates and not a single person on the island has diabetes, and not a single person was even overweight, let alone obese. Lindeberg's excellent research on the Kitavans makes it very clear that large consumption of carbohydrates does not cause overweight and obesity. [121]

Kuna: The Kuna population off the coast of Panama eats a carbohydrate-based diet that is centered around plantains, corn, cassava, kidney beans, coconuts, a variety of fruits, wild game, seafood, and chocolate. They also consume a significant amount of processed white sugar, for a total of 77 grams of sugar (unrefined and refined) per day, in addition to all the other carbohydrate-rich staple foods they consume daily. This population tends to be quite lean.[122]

Ewe Tribe in West Africa: This population eats a diet of essentially nothing but starchy tubers—about 84% carbohydrate—and is extremely lean. [123]

Hadza of Tanzania: The Hadza are one of the last hunter-gatherer populations on the planet. They eat a carbohydrate-based diet with

---

121 http://wholehealthsource.blogspot.com/2008/08/kitavans-wisdom-from-pacific-islands.html

122 http://wholehealthsource.blogspot.com/2012/06/sugar-intake-and-body-fatness-in-non.html

123 http://www.ncbi.nlm.nih.gov/pubmed/2882181

berries, baobab fruit, tubers, and honey providing the bulk of calories. Average body fat percentage among males is 11 percent, and 20 percent for females—both extremely lean by any standard.[124]

Tarahumara Indians of Mexico: This group—which is related to the Pima Indians—eats a traditional diet of mostly corn, beans, rice, potatoes, and squash, and has an extremely low incidence of type II diabetes. Their diet is 12% fat and over 75% carbohydrate.[125]

The United States: The rates of obesity in the United States have skyrocketed in the last 100 years. If we look at the USDA data from 1909-2006 on the number of calories consumed per day from protein, carbohydrates, and fat, we find something very interesting. At the beginning of the 20th century, Americans consumed a diet that was 57% carbohydrates (much of which came from white flour), and each individual was consuming about 1,400 calories per day from carbohydrates. Interestingly enough, those numbers are very close to what Americans consume today from carbohydrates.[126] In other words, the percentage of our diet that comes from carbohydrates hasn't really changed much over the last 100 years. (There have definitely been many shifts in terms of the types of carbohydrates and fats we are consuming, but in terms of overall macronutrient ratios of the diet, carbohydrate consumption has not changed dramatically over the last 100 years.) Yet, obesity rates have skyrocketed during that same time period. The only macronutrient that has actually gone up significantly during that span is our daily fat consumption.[127] Now, for those who point out that although the overall ratio of carbohydrate consumption hasn't changed, the types of carbohydrates (specifically from sugar) we are consuming has changed slightly, I would respond by pointing to two other obesity epidemics—the epidemic in the UK and that of Australia—that have both coincided with a decrease in sugar consumption and an increase in fat consumption.[128] So it's not

---

124 http://wholehealthsource.blogspot.com/2012/06/sugar-intake-and-body-fatness-in-non.html

125 http://ajcn.nutrition.org/content/32/4/905.full.pdf

126 http://wholehealthsource.blogspot.com/2011/08/carbohydrate-hypothesis-of-obesity.html

127 http://wholehealthsource.blogspot.com/2011/08/carbohydrate-hypothesis-of-obesity.html

128 http://www.mdpi.com/2072-6643/3/4/491

explainable by sugar either (as we will explore in depth in the next chapter).

So if carbohydrates are the cause of fatness, why exactly is it that carbohydrates somehow cause obesity today in the United States when they didn't 100 years ago?

And why is it that all these cultures mentioned above—many of which consume diets *higher* in carbohydrates than many populations with obesity epidemics—are lean and healthy, with negligible rates of obesity?

If carbohydrates are *the* cause of obesity, it would be incredibly easy to demonstrate such a link with very simple studies, and yet we have done these studies, and they show no evidence of such a link.

Moreover, this is not simply a case of a few studies not fitting the hypothesis. There is a mountain of data directly contradicting the hypothesis and showing that higher carbohydrate consumption has no reliable relationship to fat gain.

The simple fact is that in the traditional populations around the world that consume a high-carbohydrate diet where carbohydrates come from whole foods, diabetes, heart disease, overweight, and obesity (and other "diseases of civilization") are unheard of.

For anyone not married to the notion that carbs/insulin are evil, the obvious and inescapable conclusion from all of this is that insulin/carbohydrate/sugar consumption is not the cause of fat gain.

Debunking the Carbohydrate Theory of Obesity – Summary

To wrap all this up, we have now seen that:

- Raising insulin does not cause increased fat gain, and lowering insulin does not promote fat loss. Being on a caloric deficit while on a high-carbohydrate or low-carbohydrate diet similarly causes no difference in the amount of fat lost.
- Higher levels of insulin are indeed correlated with obesity; however, high levels of insulin are not the *cause* of obesity. But the reverse is true—obesity *does* cause higher levels of insulin—as is well known by obesity scientists. (This mistake is a good example of confusing correlation with causation.)
- Carbohydrates do not turn into fat to any significant degree that could be congruent with the Carbohydrate/Insulin Theory of Obesity. But dietary fat does and is preferentially stored as body fat in the case of a caloric excess.
- Insulin is not only released in response to eating carbohydrates, it's also released in equal and sometimes even greater amounts in response to eating many low-carb, protein-rich foods. Thus, low-carb diets fail at their most basic premise—that by avoiding carbohydrates, you will be avoiding insulin spikes.
- For insulin to actually have an impact on body fat, it would have to either increase calorie intake or decrease calorie burning. But it does neither. Insulin does not transcend basic laws of thermodynamics. There is no energy fairy.
- It is not only carbohydrates that block the burning of body fat—proteins and dietary fats will also create equivalent net storage of fat in your fat cells at the end of the day. Insulin operates within—not outside of—the calories in, calories out equation. In other words, consuming 500 calories of non-insulin-spiking fats blocks the burning of body fat just as much as consuming 500 calories of insulin-spiking carbohydrates.
- The reason some people do lose weight on low-carb diets has nothing to do with the amount of carbohydrate consumed and everything to do with the amount of protein and the amount of whole food consumed (and overall reward/palatability of the

diet). High protein intakes and whole-food diets (both of which are recommendations on nearly all low-carb diets) act to drive down total calories consumed, and this is what is really responsible for any fat loss that occurred. The same weight loss effect occurs with high-carbohydrate diets that are whole food and high-protein diets.

- Any differences that appear in non-calorie-controlled experiments of "low-carb" vs. "low-fat" diets are likely due to overall differences in total calories consumed—not due to the inherent metabolic effects of either carbs or fats. Overall calories consumed, in turn, is dictated largely by overall palatability of the diet, whole foods vs. processed foods, and protein consumption.
- Low-carb diets offer absolutely no fat loss advantage compared to higher-carb diets of equal calories and protein. When calories or protein are controlled for, the supposed benefits of low-carb diets (that show up in poorly controlled studies) completely disappear.
- Most importantly, in looking at cultures around the world, it immediately becomes clear that there is no correlation at all between the amount of carbohydrate calories eaten and body fatness. Numerous cultures around the world eat far *more* carbohydrates than we do in the United States yet have virtually undetectable rates of overweight and obesity.

Taken together, these data conclusively discredit every single tenet of the Carbohydrate Theory of Obesity. In essence, in just about every possible way that the Carbohydrate Theory of Obesity *could* be wrong, it is wrong.

Carbohydrates do not make you fat. And low-carb diets do not offer any benefit over calorie-matched and protein-matched diets with higher carbohydrates.

Fat gain and fat loss are a function of net calorie balance, not a function of the hormonal effects of dietary carbohydrate.

The Carbohydrate Theory of Obesity is now officially dead.

Chapter 3: When Food Really Does Make Us Fat - Sugar vs. Fat, Whole Foods vs. Processed Foods

So which macronutrient makes us fat—carbohydrates or fat? Trick question!

Both can be fattening, and both can also be slimming. It depends entirely on the context.

- We can find studies that implicate sugar as being fattening, but other studies contradict the notion.
- The same is true of fat—there are certainly studies that implicate fat as being fattening, while other studies contradict that finding.
- We can find studies that show eating a high-carb diet causes fat gain, and we can find studies showing that eating a high-fat diet causes fat gain.
- We can also find studies showing that eating a high-fat diet can cause fat loss and that eating a high-carb diet can cause fat loss.

Since we don't have any predictable relationship between the amount of carbs or fats a person eats (or doesn't eat) and how fat or lean they are, how can we make sense of all this seemingly contradictory data?

As a matter of fact, there is one concept—little known among most popular health and nutrition writers, but well known among obesity scientists—that can reconcile the data: **food reward/palatability.**

This is the factor that can help us make sense of this apparent conflict.

It is the single most significant and important factor to discuss when talking about how food does or doesn't make us fat.

So let's devote some time to getting into the details around this important concept.

What is Food Reward and Why Does it Matter?

If food reward/palatability is the most important factor to consider when analyzing how food makes us fat or keeps us lean, then we need to start with a basic question:

What exactly is highly rewarding, palatable food?

Well, it has been defined differently by different people, but the easiest way of understanding it is that it's food that tastes extremely good, lights up the pleasure circuitry of our brain, and stimulates us to eat *more.*

As obesity researcher Stephan Guyenet explains:

> "Food reward is the process by which eating specific foods reinforces behaviors that favor the acquisition and consumption of the food in question. You could also call rewarding food 'reinforcing' or 'habit-forming,' although not necessarily in an addictive sense. Food reward is a perfectly normal and healthy part of life, although I believe it can be harmful if it exceeds the bounds of what we're adapted to. Food reward is essential for survival in a natural environment, because it teaches you what to eat and how to get it through a trial-and-error process."[129]

Guyenet has outlined the theory, the science, and all the physiological mechanisms in his highly regarded series of articles reviewing the vast literature on the subject, so we will not go into great detail on the scientific minutiae. If you're interested in exploring the science on this in great detail, read those articles from Guyenet. Our goal here is to translate this science into simple take-home messages.

Numerous lines of research have now made it abundantly clear that food reward is a dominant factor in why people get fat—far *more* significant of a factor than the inherent metabolic effects of either carbohydrates or fat.

To make this even clearer, **food reward/palatability—*not* macronutrients—is the major factor that determines whether a given type of food is fattening or not.**

How do we know food reward is such a dominant factor in obesity?

---

129 http://wholehealthsource.blogspot.com/2011/05/food-reward-dominant-factor-in-obesity_26.html

We know this from multiple lines of evidence where researchers have shown (to paraphrase Guyenet's articles above):

1) Increasing the reward/palatability value of the diet causes fat gain in animals and humans.
2) Decreasing the reward/palatability of the diet causes fat loss in animals and humans that carry excess fat.
3) Individual sensitivity to food reward strongly predicts future fat gain.
4) Brain circuitry that controls pleasure and motivation directly interacts with other brain circuits that control food intake and body fatness.
5) Manipulation of pleasure and motivation circuits in the brain (e.g., by lesion, drugs, or genetic manipulation) affects food intake and body fatness.
6) Genetic differences that influence pleasure circuits in the brain correlate with differences in body fatness.
7) Obesity prevalence in specific societies parallels changes in the reward/palatability value of prevailing diet patterns.

These seven lines of evidence make it clear that food reward is a massive factor in fat gain. In contrast to manipulating the ratio of carbohydrate to fat—where the impact on body fatness is typically minor if present at all--manipulating the reward/palatability value of the diet has a powerful and reliable impact on body fatness. In dozens of experiments, it has been consistently shown that solely through manipulating the reward/palatability of the diet, researchers can reliably make lean animals fat and fat animals lean—all while allowing them to eat *ad libitum* (however much they want). Without restricting access to food or force feeding or changing movement/exercise habits of animals, their body fatness can be almost *completely* controlled solely through manipulating the reward/palatability value of their diet.

The science is admittedly complex, but the actual concept of this theory is relatively straightforward to the point of being basically common sense: **When you eat stuff that tastes good and makes you feel pleasure, you tend to eat *more total food* than you would have if you were eating something less tasty and pleasurable.**

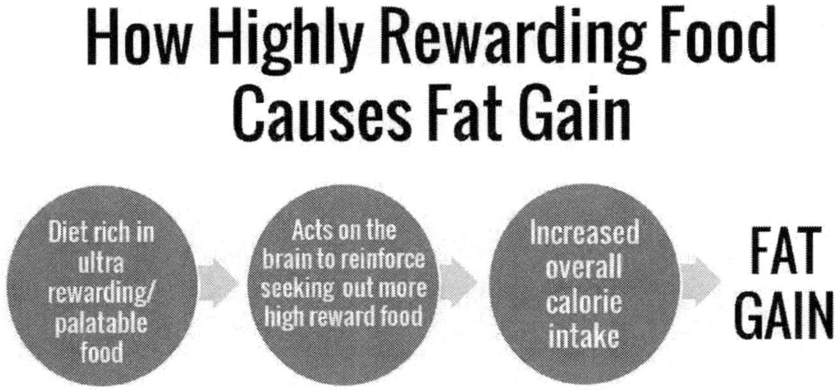
How Highly Rewarding Food Causes Fat Gain
Diet rich in ultra rewarding/ palatable food
Acts on the brain to reinforce seeking out more high reward food
Increased overall calorie intake
FAT GAIN

The way that highly rewarding food increases overall food consumption is largely due to a raising of the reward threshold in the brain. The reward threshold means the amount of a substance that is needed to feel a certain level of reward. When we have pleasurable stimuli that are in harmony with our neurological wiring, we do just fine. But when certain stimuli create excessively intense (unnaturally so) rewards, it can raise the reward threshold. This makes it so we require progressively more of a given substance to feel a certain level of reward. Just as this effect is problematic when it occurs with harmful drugs, it is also problematic when this effect starts happening with food.

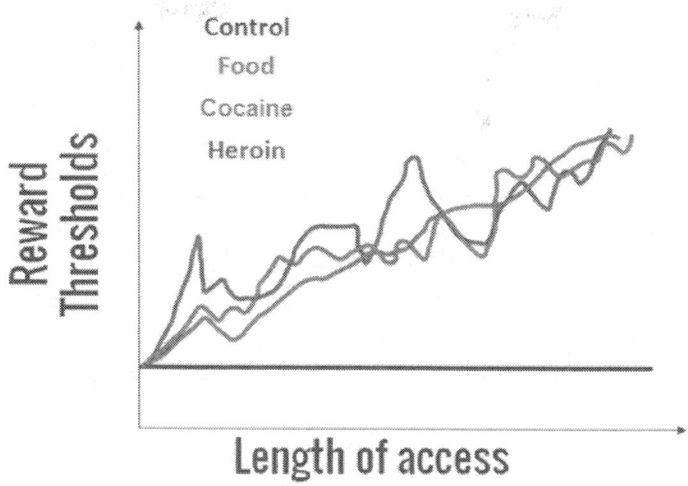

(Source: Modeled after the graph in the study "Reward Mechanisms in Obesity: New Insights and Future Directions"[130])

As the reward threshold goes up, so too do our consumption of highly rewarding food and overall calories.

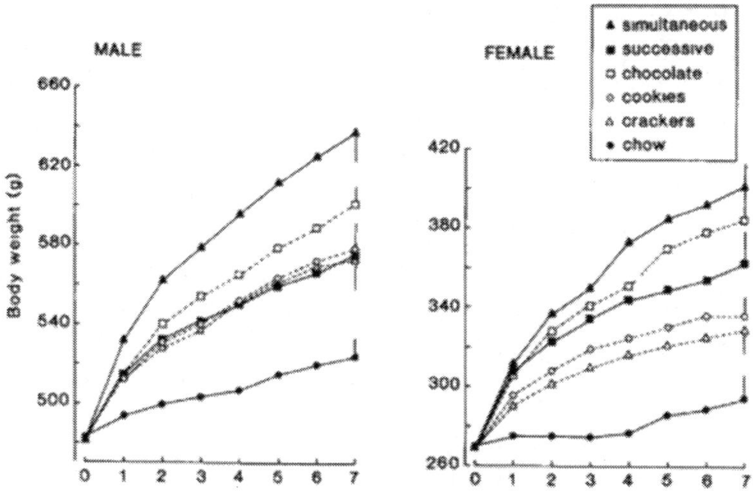

(Source: Stephan Guyenet. Why Do We Overeat? A Neurobiological Perspective.)

130 http://www.ncbi.nlm.nih.gov/pmc/articles/PMC3057652/

As this experiment shows, as we have continued access to highly rewarding food, we tend to consume more overall calories and thus get fatter. The more rewarding the food we have access to, the fatter we tend to become.

In direct contrast to the paucity of evidence suggesting that carbohydrates are a major factor in fat gain, there is currently a body of over 3,000 studies on the subject of reward/palatability and body fatness, and this body of evidence has made it extremely clear that reward/palatability is a dominant factor in the obesity epidemic. As has been corroborated by numerous comprehensive literature reviews, **the evidence is simply overwhelming that extremely *palatable and rewarding* food—rather than any specific nutrient—is the major nutrition-related cause of fat gain.**

- From the literature review titled **"Modulation of taste responsiveness and food preference by obesity and weight loss":** "Palatable foods lead to overeating, and it is almost a forgone conclusion that it is also an important contributor to the current obesity epidemic—there is even talk about food addiction." [131]
- From the literature review titled **"Food reward, hyperphagia, and obesity":** "Given the unabated obesity problem, there is increasing appreciation of expressions like 'my eyes are bigger than my stomach,' and recent studies in rodents and humans suggest that dysregulated brain reward pathways may be contributing not only to drug addiction but also to increased intake of palatable foods and ultimately obesity."[132]
- From the literature review titled **"Neural mechanisms underlying obesity and drug addiction":** "Increasing rates of obesity have alarmed health officials and prompted much public dialogue. While the factors leading to obesity are numerous, an inability to control intake of freely available food is central to the problem." [133]
- From the literature review titled **"Dual roles of dopamine in food and drug seeking: the drive-reward paradox":** "That

131 http://www.ncbi.nlm.nih.gov/pubmed/22521912

132 http://www.ncbi.nlm.nih.gov/pubmed/21411768

133 http://www.ncbi.nlm.nih.gov/pubmed/17292426

the same brain circuitry is implicated in the motivation for and the reinforcement by both food and addictive drugs extends the argument for a common mechanism underlying compulsive overeating and compulsive drug taking."[134]

- From the literature review titled **"The contribution of brain reward circuits to the obesity epidemic":** "We discuss contemporary research that suggests that hyperphagia leading to obesity is associated with substantial neurochemical changes in the brain. These findings verify the relevance of reward pathways for promoting consumption of palatable, calorically dense foods, and lead to the important question of whether changes in reward circuitry in response to intake of such foods serve a causal role in the development and maintenance of some cases of obesity. We suggest that it might be more useful to focus on overeating that results in frank obesity, and multiple health, interpersonal, and occupational negative consequences as a form of food 'abuse.'"[135]
- From the literature review titled **"Dopamine signaling in food addiction: role of dopamine D2 receptors":** "Recent evidence now suggests that as with drug addiction, obesity with compulsive eating behaviors involves reward circuitry of the brain, particularly the circuitry involving dopaminergic neural substrates. Increasing amounts of data from human imaging studies, together with genetic analysis, have demonstrated that obese people and drug addicts tend to show altered expression of DA D2 receptors in specific brain areas, and that similar brain areas are activated by food-related and drug-related cues." [136]
- Finally, we have a massively important and comprehensive work from renowned obesity scientist Rudolph Leibel, MD, among other scientists, titled **"Obesity and Leptin Resistance: Distinguishing Cause from Effect,"** which states: "While genetic alterations in humans and animals have taught us a great deal about mechanisms of severe obesity and

134 http://www.ncbi.nlm.nih.gov/pubmed/23044182

135 http://www.ncbi.nlm.nih.gov/pubmed/23237885

136 http://www.ncbi.nlm.nih.gov/pmc/articles/PMC4133846/

> the systems that govern energy balance, **it appears that the changed environment, not altered genetics, underlies the burgeoning epidemic of obesity in developed and developing countries. During the last 50 years, two major changes have shifted the energy balance equation: the decreased requirement for physical energy expenditure and the increased availability and abundance of palatable, calorically dense foods. A common research model of obesity investigators, diet-induced obesity (DIO), mirrors the ubiquity of highly palatable calorie-dense foods in modern societies.** In this paradigm, animals remain lean when maintained on standard chow, but increase their caloric intake and rapidly gain adipose mass when provided a calorically dense diet (generally high in both fat and sugar content). **While genetic predispositions to DIO clearly exist (some rodent strains gain little weight on high-calorie compared to normal chow, while others rapidly progress to obesity), it is the availability of a highly palatable diet that drives overeating and subsequent obesity in these models."**[137]

It is also worth noting that this theory makes it clear that overeating is *not* a simple matter of gluttony and sloth (i.e., a simple case of "eating too many calories" whereby the solution is as simple as "count calories and eat fewer of them"). Rather, it is calorie overconsumption driven by non-conscious neurological and hormonal influences driving us to consume more calories.

Thus, rather than trying to evaluate whether low-fat or low-carb is the best (i.e., trying to find the value of the diet in the inherent metabolic effects of fats or carbohydrates), as the nutrition discussion has been directed in the United States for the last several decades, we ought to be framing a discussion of what type of diet is fattening in the context of food reward and palatability. This would be infinitely more instructive and useful than this silly approach of trying to blame the world's ills on a single food group and then adopting ideologies based on that premise (e.g., low carb, vegan, low fat).

---

137 http://www.ncbi.nlm.nih.gov/pmc/articles/PMC2967652/

So if food reward/palatability is such a dominant factor in obesity, then the most important question to ask is, "What kinds of foods are the most rewarding/palatable?"

Generally speaking, modern processed industrial food products are the most rewarding/palatable. More specifically, it is processed foods with a dense combination of refined sugars and fats (often mixed with artificial flavorings) that are professionally engineered to maximize the reward factor in the brain and surpass the brain's natural reward threshold.

Importantly, food reward/palatability is *not* an effect unique to either carbohydrates/sugar or fat. Sugar by itself is not especially rewarding, though it is moderately so. Fat by itself is not especially rewarding, though it is moderately so.

When in the context of nearly all whole, natural foods, these are rewarding stimuli within the bounds of the brain's reward threshold, and thus, whole-food sugars and fats tend not to be fattening.

But combine fats and sugars in a highly concentrated end-product that would never occur in a natural food (say in the form of ice cream, or pie with cream on top), and lace the combination with a bunch of artificial flavorings that are professionally engineered with the specific intent to maximize the fireworks in the pleasure center of the brain, and, well, you have extraordinarily rewarding food. You have a superstimuli effect that will surpass the brain's tolerance for reward. Over time, this drives you to continually consume more of the substance.

When you eat highly rewarding food frequently, it's likely that you'll have a hard time getting enough of the stuff.

When you eat a diet composed largely of highly rewarding, processed food, it disrupts the body's ability to regulate energy balance (calories in, calories out) normally, and instead of eating because your body requires fuel, you start eating in order to give yourself neurological pleasure. Your eating behaviors become *progressively dissociated from eating according to your body's biological need.* As a result of eating to give yourself neurological pleasure, you become numb to the signals telling you to stop eating and instead start listening to your brain's cravings for more pleasure, which, over time, tend to drive you to eat beyond your body's biological need. Essentially, what's going on is that the hedonic system in your brain is *overriding* the brain's normal tendency to regulate appetite in accordance with calorie burning. You start craving food for want of pleasure rather than need of fuel. Naturally, this leads to chronic calorie overconsumption and fat gain.

But again, it's not that processed food is mechanistically more fattening because it turns to fat more easily or something due to its inherent metabolic effects—it's that, over time, highly rewarding food disrupts the energy regulation center of the brain in such a way that you end up chronically overconsuming calories.

Fat vs. Carbs: Which is the Most Fattening?

Now that we've established that excessively rewarding food—rather than the inherent hormonal effects of any macronutrient in particular—is the major factor that dictates whether the diet is fattening or not, we can still go back to the question of fat versus carbs. But now we've shifted the frame of the argument: the argument is now framed in the context of food reward/palatability and which of these two macronutrients—fat or carbs—is more rewarding, and thus more likely to drive up calorie intake and be fattening.

One variation on the theme of blaming the obesity epidemic on carbohydrates is that carbohydrates don't necessarily make you fatter due to their inherent metabolic effects (e.g., "insulin causes fat storage"), but they cause you to eat more, and therefore make you fatter by making you eat more total calories. This is often stated as something like, "Carbs spike your blood sugar and then it comes crashing back down, which stimulates you to eat *even more* carbs, which puts you into a vicious cycle of constantly eating more and more, and thus, getting fatter" or that "fats are more satiating than carbs—when you eat carbs, you just crave more carbs and end up eating more." According to this logic, even if equal amounts of carbohydrate calories aren't inherently more fattening, carbohydrates are still to blame for the obesity epidemic because a carbohydrate-rich eating style increases food intake, which makes you fatter.

For those intent on seeing things through the lens of macronutrients, the question is now this: How does the palatability/reward of carbs compare to fat? Which of these two macronutrients really drives up our calorie consumption the most?

Fortunately, the theory often heard from low-carb gurus that carbohydrate/sugar consumption drives us to eat more calories more powerfully than fats has actually been tested in numerous studies.

The research is extremely clear that carbohydrates and sugars are not uniquely fattening and that carbohydrates do not drive up calorie intake to a greater degree than fat-rich diets do.

For example, here are a few quotes from the studies on the subject:

- **"Foods high in dietary fat have a weak effect on satiation, which leads to a form of passive overconsumption, and a disproportionately weak effect on satiety (joule-for-joule**

compared with protein and carbohydrate). This overconsumption (high-fat hyperphagia) is dependent upon both the high energy density and the potent sensory qualities (high palatability) of high-fat foods."[138]

- "LF [low-fat], lower-energy diets are more satiating than are HF [high-fat], higher-energy diets, but carbohydrate stores per se did not entirely account for the change that diet composition had on energy intake. This study suggests that protein and carbohydrate have potential to reduce subsequent energy intake whereas there was no apparent reductive effect due to fat."
- Another study specifically found that high fat intake in meals actually decreases satiety in obese people (by suppressing the hunger hormone ghrelin less effectively than carbohydrates) and promotes calorie overconsumption: "These results suggest that impaired ghrelin response after HF meals may contribute to reduced satiety and overeating, especially among obese individuals."[139]
- A study titled "The Role of Energy Density in the Overconsumption of Fat" stated: "In recent years, research has focused on why fat is so readily overconsumed. Although the palatability of many high-fat foods can encourage overconsumption, another possibility is that fat is not very satiating. **A number of studies have compared the effects of fat and carbohydrate on both satiation (the amount eaten in a meal) and satiety (the effect on subsequent intake), but have found little difference between these macronutrients when the palatability and energy density were similar. On the other hand, the energy density of foods has been demonstrated to have a robust and significant effect on both satiety and satiation, independently of palatability and macronutrient content. It is likely that the high energy density of many high-fat foods facilitates the overconsumption of fat."**[140]

---

138 http://www.ncbi.nlm.nih.gov/pubmed/9216571

139 http://www.ncbi.nlm.nih.gov/pubmed/19458028

140 http://jn.nutrition.org/content/130/2/268.full.pdf

When ad libitum diets (diets where calories are not limited and people can eat however much they desire) high in carbohydrates are compared to diets high in fat, the studies tend to indicate that, at best, high-fat diets are equally satiating as high-carbohydrate diets, and, at worst, higher-fat diets are less satiating and *more fattening*.[141] [142] [143] [144] [145] [146]

Overall, the data actually shows us that if anything, high-fat diets are likely slightly *more* palatable/rewarding than high-carb diets!

As Guyenet showed in his comprehensive literature review, [147] we see this effect of high-fat diets being more fattening than high-carb diets in both short-term studies,[148] [149] [150] [151] [152] as well as longer-term studies. [153] [154] [155] [156] [157]

The science bears out this conclusion over and over again—diets higher in fats tend to drive calorie overconsumption and fat gain *more* than diets high in carbohydrates.

Also worth noting here is the effect on satiety, since many low-carb advocates like to claim that eating fat "makes you feel full" and thus causes you to eat less. Contrary to popular belief, fat is not particularly

141 http://www.ncbi.nlm.nih.gov/pubmed/9216571

142 http://www.ncbi.nlm.nih.gov/pubmed/3687822

143 http://www.ncbi.nlm.nih.gov/pubmed/7625338

144 http://www.ncbi.nlm.nih.gov/pubmed/10682875

145 http://www.ncbi.nlm.nih.gov/pubmed/2021123

146 http://www.ncbi.nlm.nih.gov/pubmed/1570800

147 http://wholehealthsource.blogspot.com/2014/06/calorie-intake-and-body-fatness-on-high.html

148 http://www.ncbi.nlm.nih.gov/pubmed/9280170

149 http://www.ncbi.nlm.nih.gov/pubmed/8475895

150 http://ajcn.nutrition.org/content/62/2/330.short

151 http://ajcn.nutrition.org/content/62/2/316.short

152 http://www.ncbi.nlm.nih.gov/pubmed/8395476

153 http://www.ncbi.nlm.nih.gov/pubmed/9216571

154 http://www.ncbi.nlm.nih.gov/pubmed/3687822

155 http://www.ncbi.nlm.nih.gov/pubmed/7625338

156 http://www.ncbi.nlm.nih.gov/pubmed/10682875

157 http://www.ncbi.nlm.nih.gov/pubmed/2021123

satiating (as the above studies clearly show), and added fats/oils are generally quite effective at driving up overall calorie consumption with little increase in satiety. Protein is by far the most satiating macronutrient, while fat and carbohydrates are roughly equally as satiating.

This fattening effect of added fats is obviously strongest with diets high in refined foods (which are higher reward diets), but it does occur to some extent with adding fats to unrefined diets. For example, just think about eating raw dry kale leaves by themselves as opposed to adding some oil or cheese on top of them—which one is more palatable? Obviously, with the oil or cheese, they become tremendously more palatable than just the raw kale leaves by themselves. Thus, adding that fat causes you to eat many more calories than you would have if you were just eating the plain leaves. Adding the fat doesn't increase satiety and make you eat less overall calories—to the contrary, it causes *increased* calorie consumption. And if you doubt the validity of this comparison, we ask you to consider how "addictive" eating fatty, low-carb foods like cheese and peanut butter can be. How often have you found yourself not being able to put the jar of peanut butter down? Clearly, very fatty, low-carb foods can drive up calorie consumption as well or more than carbohydrate-rich foods.

As the above studies show, fat can drive up calorie consumption as much or more than carbohydrate.[158] Note that all of this research is ignored by advocates of low-carb, high-fat diets who like to claim that it is specifically carbohydrates that drive calorie overconsumption, with claims like "fat doesn't make you fat, sugar does" and "fat satiates you and gives you steady energy, while carbs spike your insulin and cause you to crash, which makes you hungry for more sugar and causes you to eat even more." All of these claims are utter pseudoscience that is directly contradicted by the research. A high-*protein* diet is certainly satiating (and such claims could legitimately be made about high-protein diets), but there just aren't significant differences in satiety or food intake on carbohydrate-based diets compared to fat-based diets. And if any argument is to be made, it is that fat is the more fattening macronutrient.

---

158 http://wholehealthsource.blogspot.com/2014/06/calorie-intake-and-body-fatness-on-high.html

The simple truth is that the recommendations from scientists during the 1980s and 1990s to eat lower-fat diets actually had a sound basis in science. Not because "fat makes you fat" by virtue of its inherent metabolic effects, but because high-fat diets promote higher calorie intakes, and because reducing a major food group from the diet (fats, in this case) is an effective means of reducing overall calorie intake and causing fat loss. Moreover, "low-fat" and "no-fat" processed junk foods had not been created by the food industry at that time, and thus the recommendations to eat a low-fat diet were not intended to make us all switch from fatty foods to processed junk full of refined grains and sugars, but to get us to switch to eating more fruits, vegetables, and plant foods. And that is a low-fat dietary pattern that *does* have proven anti-obesity effects.

As it turns out, the typical low-carb guru claim that those scientists who told us to eat lower-fat diets were a bunch of idiots (or were deliberately misrepresenting the science) has no basis in reality. In fact, research was quite clear that low-fat dietary interventions were indeed an effective way of lowering overall calorie intake and causing fat loss. (Again, removal of any major food group or macronutrient—like fats or carbs—from the diet results in lowering the palatability/reward of the diet, thereby spontaneously decreasing food intake and causing weight loss. Low-fat and low-carb diets work the same way in this regard.)

The bottom line is that, in the context of diets that are not calorie matched, fats can indeed drive fat gain by enhancing palatability and food reward—as much or *more* than carbohydrates do.

Overall, the research shows us that dietary fat is likely just as palatable/rewarding (and thus, just as fattening) as carbohydrates are.

This is why most studies indicate that low-carb and low-fat diets (when matched for protein intake) tend to be about equally as effective for weight loss in the long term.[159]

---

159 http://www.ncbi.nlm.nih.gov/pubmed/25182101

The Two Potential Dietary Culprits for Obesity: Sugar and Fat

The USDA data indicates that perhaps the two most significant potential culprits in the food supply for this increase in calorie consumption over the last 100 years (coinciding with the obesity epidemic of the last 50 years or so) are the increase in added sugars and added fats to the diet. Let's take a closer look at each of these:

1) The increase in added sugars.

Since 1909, refined sugar consumption has increased by 74.9%.[160] (Note that overall carbohydrate content of the diet did not increase significantly, since the sugars displaced other sources of carbohydrate.)

If we go back further in time, the increase in sugar consumption is even more staggering. There is simply no doubt that sugar consumption has increased dramatically since it was first manufactured on a large scale in the 1800s:

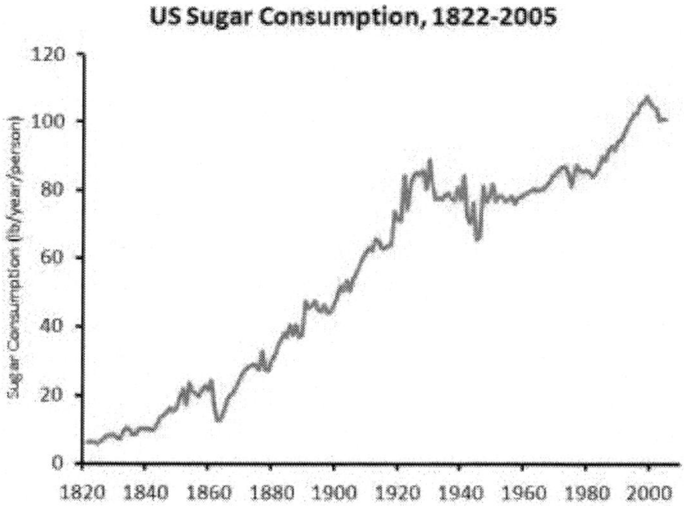

160 http://www.cnpp.usda.gov/sites/default/files/nutrient_content_of_the_us_food_supply/FoodSupply1909-2000.pdf

But before you rush to assume that this is the cause of the obesity epidemic, consider that while the obesity epidemic in the United States has coincided with an increase in sugar consumption, both the UK and Australian obesity epidemics have actually coincided with a decrease in sugar consumption. (More on this later in this chapter.)

2) The increase in added fats.

Since 1909, consumption of shortening increased 200%, consumption of margarine increased 800%, and consumption of salad and cooking oils increased by 1,450%. [161] (Note that overall fat consumption also increased significantly over the last century.)

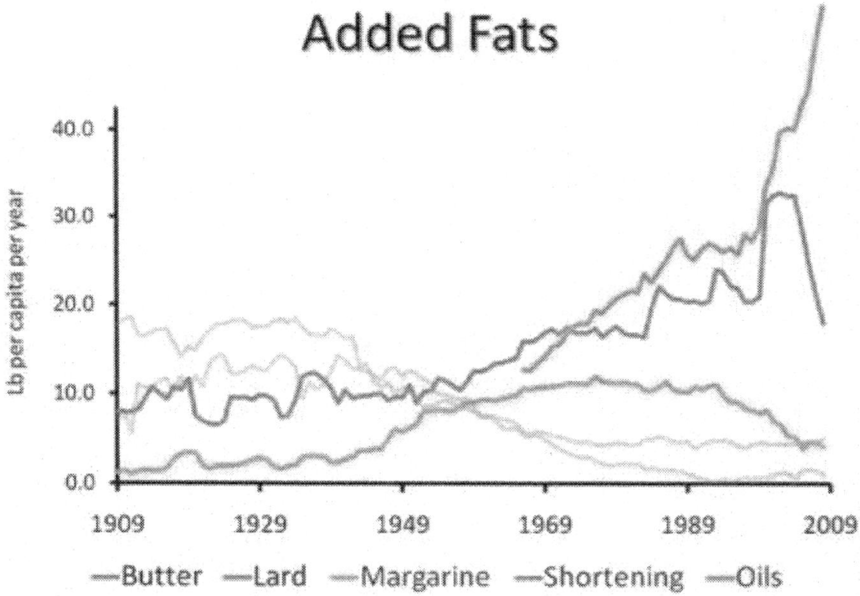

Here you can see how consumption of shortening and vegetable oil consumption skyrocketed before and during the obesity epidemic. (Source: Stephan Guyenet. The American Diet. *2012.).*

161 http://www.cnpp.usda.gov/sites/default/files/nutrient_content_of_the_us_food_supply/FoodSupply1909-2000.pdf

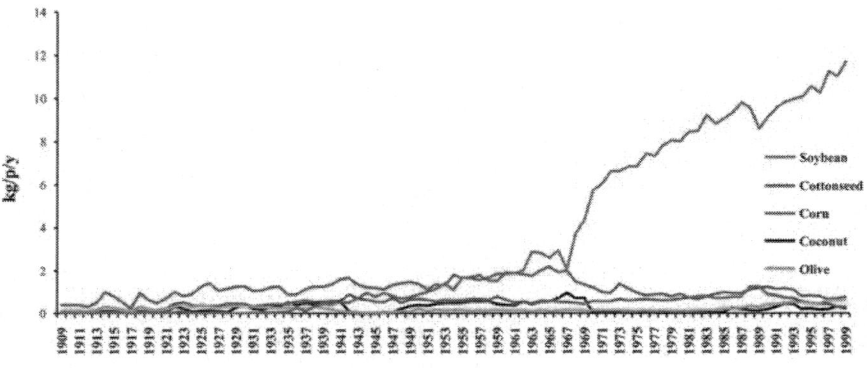

Here you can see how consumption of soybean oil has become a major contributor to the overall calories consumed each day by most Americans. As of 1999, soybean oil alone comprises 7% of the calories consumed by Americans, which is enormous.[162]

In terms of linking specific changes in the food supply with the obesity epidemic, the increase in added fats and added sugars are the two most obvious potential culprits.

But while many people have sought to reduce the obesity epidemic down to a matter of the inherent metabolic effects of one or the other of these two nutrients (i.e., the low-fat movement and the low-carb movement), we are suggesting to you that neither is correct.

Both added sugars and added fats have played a role in the obesity epidemic—but not as a result of their inherent metabolic effects. This is *not* a case of fat making us fat because "fat makes you fat," nor is this a case of "carbs and sugars make us fat because of the insulin." Both of these notions are simply wrong. Rather, ***both added sugars and fats*** **have contributed to the epidemic by raising the overall reward/palatability value in the food supply and causing us to consume more calories overall.**

This is *not* due to the inherent metabolic or hormonal effects of either sugar or fat, or of some inherent metabolic effects of processed foods—it's due to the *taste* and *neurological reward* effects causing us to simply eat *more total calories* than we did previously when we were eating simpler, less processed, less palatable, and less rewarding whole foods.

---

162 http://ajcn.nutrition.org/content/93/5/950.short

Obesity epidemics can occur and worsen with a wide range of macronutrient profiles in the diet, and they *do not* depend upon the inherent metabolic effects of either sugar or fat *per se*. What they *do* depend on is ample consumption of highly rewarding processed food.

How Can You Be So Sure that Sugar Doesn't Make Us Fat Due to its Inherent Metabolic/Hormonal Effects?

By now, it should be clear to you that there is nothing inherently fattening about carbohydrates or insulin. The amount of carbohydrates in your diet and the amount of insulin your body produces after you eat are simply not related in any meaningful way to how much body fat your body stores.

So you might be wondering, "Okay, well maybe carbs *per se* aren't fattening, but maybe sugar is?!"

So let's talk about sugar! Sugar has certainly been demonized extensively by just about everyone in the nutrition world with everything from "sugar causes diabetes" to "sugar is a toxic poison" to "fat doesn't make you fat, sugar does."

First, let's define what sugar is.

In this section, we use the word "sugar" to refer to three things: 1) sucrose, or table sugar, 2) high-fructose corn syrup (HFCS), and 3) fruit and honey sugars (and fruit juices, maple syrup, etc.).

Sucrose = one molecule of glucose and one molecule of fructose linked together, and it is therefore 50:50 glucose:fructose. When you eat sucrose, this bond is rapidly broken, releasing free glucose and fructose, which are then absorbed.

HFCS = mixture of free glucose and fructose that comes in two common varieties: 42:55 and 53:42 glucose:fructose. The former is most often used in soft drinks, while the latter is most often used in baked goods. (Note: Since sucrose and HFCS are both refined sugars composed of roughly half glucose, half fructose, one would expect them to have similar effects on the body, and overall, controlled experiments have confirmed that they do.)

Fruit Sugar = mixture of sucrose, free glucose, and free fructose.

Honey = composed of roughly half free fructose and half free glucose.

So what's the deal—is sugar (or any of the different types of sugar) inherently fattening?

As already shown in earlier sections, in metabolic ward studies where people are put on either high- or low-carb diets of equal calories, they achieve precisely equal amounts of fat gain or fat loss.

But what happens when you do the same experiments with sugar specifically? Is a given number of calories from sugar more fattening than from other nutrients?

- Rodriguez et al. conducted a study where obese women were put on a diet with high levels of natural sugar (fruit) or low levels of natural sugar on equal-calorie diets for eight weeks. The study concluded that both groups had essentially the same amount of weight loss and similar improvement of markers of metabolic health: "The induced weight loss was similar for both diets (6.9 +/- 2% vs. 6.6 +/- 2%, p = 0.785). Both experimental diets similarly improved the lipid plasma profile in the participants, but the cholesterol fall was higher in obese subjects receiving the diet containing more fruit."[163]
- Now, if we do basically the same study but use refined sugar, maybe the result will turn out differently? Surwit and colleagues conducted a study to find out. They compared the six-week effects of two diets that consisted of identical total calories, but one had 43% of the total calories as sucrose (table sugar), and one had only 4% of the total calories as sucrose.[164] Here again, we see the exact same result: no significant differences were seen in the loss of body weight or body fat between the high- and low-sucrose groups.

Let us emphasize here that the above study did not use sugar from whole natural foods, but refined white table sugar. And still, no difference in weight loss.

So immediately we can see that the low-carb gurus are wrong about sugar: sugar is ***not*** inherently fattening. **Equal calorie diets, whether high or low in sugar, will result in equal weight gain or weight loss.**

This is, of course, consistent with all of the research we have already shown you that proves that insulin spikes from carbohydrate-

---

163 http://www.ncbi.nlm.nih.gov/pubmed/16395633

164 http://www.ncbi.nlm.nih.gov/pubmed/9094871

containing meals are simply *not* a significant factor in how much fat your body has on it.

There is nothing—we repeat, *nothing*—inherently fattening about sugar.

When Sugar Makes You Fat, and When Sugar Makes you *Lean*

In the last section, we looked at calorie-controlled experiments that are either high or low in sugar and found no difference in weight loss, showing that sugar is not inherently fattening due to its metabolic effects (i.e., insulin).

But we've also told you that added sugars can indeed raise the overall reward value of the diet and promote increased calorie consumption and fat gain in some contexts (on par with the potency of added fats).

So the question is this: When is sugar fattening, and when is it not fattening?

This is where things get confusing because, depending on the study you look at and the *type* of sugary foods consumed (whether the sugar is coming from whole foods or refined foods), you will find that sugar has remarkably different effects.

Believe it or not, the research on sugar is not nearly as cut and dried as the frequent demonization of it by popular health gurus and the media would suggest. **The studies are all over the place, with some suggesting high-sugar diets are fattening and others showing that high-sugar diets do not necessarily cause fat gain and can even cause fat *loss!***

Here is a brief sampling of the relevant research on sugar, showing the huge variance in outcomes:

Animal studies - In general, animal studies show mixed results in terms of the fattening effect of sugar. In rodents, some types of sugary diets can be fattening (relative to starch),[165] [166] [167] but in other cases, sugary diets can be slimming relative to starch.[168] [169] [170] [171]

---

165 http://www.ncbi.nlm.nih.gov/pubmed/8946441

166 http://www.ncbi.nlm.nih.gov/pubmed/833676

167 http://www.ncbi.nlm.nih.gov/pubmed/433810

168 http://www.ncbi.nlm.nih.gov/pubmed/10063624

169 http://www.ncbi.nlm.nih.gov/pubmed/3670072

170 http://www.ncbi.nlm.nih.gov/pubmed/9826212

171 http://www.ncbi.nlm.nih.gov/pubmed/7752914

Sugar-sweetened beverages - In general, sugar-sweetened beverages promote fat gain. In humans, we know that sugar-sweetened beverages are consistently linked with higher body fatness.[172] [173] And we have numerous other studies and meta-analyses that link consumption of sugar-sweetened beverages with higher body fatness.[174] This is well known and not controversial.

Purified fructose added to liquids - This likely promotes fat gain but is not a major factor in obesity. Very high levels of consumption of refined fructose, mostly from sweetened beverages and food, is associated with higher levels of visceral (belly) fat in US adolescents but is not associated with total body fatness.[175] The most recent review of the effects of fructose (as of June 2014) failed to implicate fructose consumption as a causal factor in the obesity epidemic.[176]

Bland liquids - Numerous other studies and meta-analyses have concluded that sugar is not fattening in many contexts, such as when consumed in whole foods and/or in bland liquids. Some studies have shown that sugar-rich beverages can even be used as weight loss shakes! In fact, one scientific review from the *American Journal of Clinical Nutrition*, when speaking about sugar-containing meal replacement beverages, notes, "Numerous clinical studies have shown that sugar-containing liquids, when consumed in place of usual meals, can lead to a significant and sustained weight loss."[177]

Whole-food sugars - Numerous studies with some kinds of high-sugar diets where the sugar is derived from whole foods have shown remarkable amounts of fat loss! (These studies will be explored in detail in the next section.)

---

172 http://www.sciencedirect.com/science/article/pii/S0140673600040411

173 http://ajcn.nutrition.org/content/84/2/274.short

174 http://www.ncbi.nlm.nih.gov/pmc/articles/PMC3210834/

175 http://www.ncbi.nlm.nih.gov/pubmed/22190023

176 http://www.ncbi.nlm.nih.gov/pubmed/24666553

177 http://www.ncbi.nlm.nih.gov/pubmed/17344485

If we were forced to form some sort of overarching statement that summarizes the effects of sugar related to body fat, it would be what Guyenet says here:

> **"Overall, the observational evidence suggests that sugar in the form of sugar-sweetened beverages is associated with elevated body fatness, but total sugar intake is not."**[178]

In general, if we lump every kind of sugar (refined vs. unrefined/whole-food sugars, and sugar-containing beverages vs. sugars not in beverage form) all under the simplistic umbrella term "sugar" in order to see "the effects of sugar," there is simply no clear pattern that emerges. Some studies indicate that it is fattening, and others show that it's not only not fattening, but may actually be *slimming*.

Now, of course, it is possible to cherry-pick the data to support either the notion that sugar is perfectly healthy and not fattening (as certain dietary ideologues do, like followers of Ray Peat) or the opposite stance that sugar is terribly unhealthy and extremely fattening (like many low-carb advocates do). However, neither of these is an accurate position, and to take either position is a misrepresentation of the research.

Depending on where the sugar comes from, it has radically different effects.

Thus, it is not possible to talk about this subject intelligently so long as one insists on talking about "sugar" as if it were all one thing regardless of the source and always has the same ultimate effects on the body (as most people and most health gurus unfortunately do). This is a plainly stupid and ignorant way of discussing this subject that will lead one endlessly in confusing, unproductive directions.

Any discussion about the effects of sugar on the body must be grounded in the context of where those sugars are coming from. Otherwise, the discussion is guaranteed to be inaccurate nonsense. We'll see why that is so important in a moment, but for now, the important thing to realize is that the research, overall, certainly does *not* suggest that sugar is inherently fattening.

When the entirety of the research is considered, it shows that sometimes eating a high-sugar diet causes fat gain, sometimes

---

178 http://wholehealthsource.blogspot.com/2012/02/is-sugar-fattening.html

it doesn't cause fat gain, and sometimes it actually causes *fat loss.*

How is this possible?

The reason this is the case is because the overall effect of the sugar—whether it is fattening or slimming—is *not* dictated by the inherent metabolic effects of the sugar itself. It's about the food that sugar is consumed in!

It's Not About the Sugar Itself; the Effect is Dictated by the Package the Sugar Comes In

The potential for sugar to be fattening can come from a couple of factors:

1) Calorie to Satiety Ratio: Sugar consumed in beverage form may not promote satiety as well as solid foods and thus may lead to passive overconsumption of calories by virtue of the calorie to satiety ratio being so high. With such an unnaturally high energy density—like is seen in many processed industrial sugar-sweetened beverages—it simply becomes possible to consume very large amounts of calories before feeling satiated. This is likely why sugar-sweetened beverages are consistently linked to fat gain, while overall sugar consumption is not.
2) Palatability/Food Reward: As you will see in the next several sections, the fattening effect of sugar is primarily dependent on the palatability and reward of the package it comes in, not the inherent metabolic effects of sugar molecules.

In simple terms, if the sugar in your diet comes in the form of foods that are extremely calorie dense or food that tastes unnaturally delicious, it will tend to be fattening.

This is a big shift in paradigm from the way many people normally think about sugar. Sugar is *not* inherently fattening relative to any other nutrient, like starch or fat. There is no inherent fattening effect that results from the metabolic effects of sugar molecules. They don't turn into fat more easily or cause your body to be in "fat-storage mode" or cause an "insulin spike that makes your body store fat" or any other such nonsense.

Rather, *some types of sugar-containing foods* can be fattening by virtue of the simple fact that eating things that are extremely pleasurable and palatable tend to drive us to eat *more overall calories* than we would if we were eating something that wasn't quite as pleasurable.

- In general, eating a high-sugar diet where the sugar is coming from whole foods, like fruit, will, *at the very least,* not make you any fatter. If you're overweight and currently eating ample processed food, eating a large portion of your diet as sugar-rich whole foods will likely make you *leaner.* This is because the sugar is coming in a package (whole, unprocessed foods) that is compatible with our brain reward and satiety mechanisms. This sugar does not, in any way, promote increased calorie consumption or fat gain. Numerous studies have verified this.

- Sugars that are stripped from the whole foods they were derived from and then added into or on top of other foods will, in general, tend to cause increased consumption of overall calories, which will promote fat gain. This happens with sugar-sweetened beverages like soda and other sugar-sweetened beverages, and likely with refined sugars added on top of foods (e.g., cinnamon rolls, cakes, cookies, doughnuts, etc.).

What explains this contrast—why would sugar have such different effects depending on the package it's consumed in?

The factor that makes sense of this is food reward/palatability.

If the sugar does not taste particularly incredible—that is, if it is not *unnaturally* tasty—it will tend to drive you to eat the same amount or even fewer calories, thus maintaining your weight or causing weight loss, respectively.

But if the sugar is ingested in a way that tastes especially wonderful, it will tend to drive you to eat more overall calories, and thus contribute to fat gain.

(Note also, for any low-carb gurus seeking to demonize sugar, that added refined *fats have the exact same effect.* This is not something unique to sugar or carbohydrates, and the effect isn't dependent upon insulin or anything unique to carbohydrates. It is driven by food that's highly palatable and is rewarding in the brain—and both sugars and fats do that. We'll look at studies that directly compare the reward/palatability of sugar versus fat in a moment.)

Again, the key factor in determining whether sugar is fattening or not is taste/palatability.

But how do we really know that the fattening effects of sugar are due to palatability or whether they really are dependent on the inherent metabolic effects of sugar?

Well, aside from the calorie-matched studies we already looked at that compared high-sugar and low-sugar diets of equal calories, there is one other particularly brilliant way to test whether the fattening effect of sugar is due to its inherent metabolic effects, or whether it's due to the sweet taste simply stimulating you to eat more calories: compare the effects of sugar in animals that have the ability to taste sweetness and those that don't.

Interestingly enough, this experiment has been done! The study asked a simple question: **Is sugar still fattening if one can't taste its sweetness?**

They took rodents and genetically "knocked out" two different proteins that are required for the perception of sweet tastes on the tongue itself.

Amazingly, when the mice can't taste sweetness, the mice become almost completely resistant to the fattening effects of sugar, despite consuming a similar amount of sugar. **When they couldn't taste the sweetness, they didn't get fat!**

To test the results further and ensure that these mice weren't somehow resistant to fat gain in general, the researchers then added a small amount of fat to the water solution that the mice were drinking. Sure enough, the mice that couldn't taste sweetness (and thus didn't get fat on the sugar solution) all of the sudden became fat when given access to the solution containing fat.

They concluded that sugar *does* need to be tasted as sweet in order for it to be fattening: **"Our results suggest that nutritive solutions must be highly palatable to cause carbohydrate-induced obesity in mice..."**[179] [180]

That's the key to understanding sugar. It's not the inherent metabolic effects of sugar molecules—it's largely the taste. Delicious tasting food tends to cause us to eat more overall calories.

And importantly, either sugar or fat can increase the palatability enough to drive overconsumption of calories!

This is a rodent study, which critics will point out as a limitation. However, this result is consistent with numerous lines of human evidence. In humans, sweet tastes in the *absence* of any sugar whatsoever—like with artificial sweeteners—can be fattening via this same mechanism. While not all research is consistent with this

---

179 http://www.ncbi.nlm.nih.gov/pubmed/22683548

180 http://wholehealthsource.blogspot.com/2012/06/new-study-demonstrates-that-sugar-has.html

outcome,[181] a great deal of research shows that in non-calorie-controlled settings, artificial sweeteners (which have none of the metabolic effects of sugar) can be equally as fattening as sugar, and sometimes, even more fattening.[182] [183] [184] [185] [186] [187] [188] So here we can see the result of completely uncoupling sweetness with the metabolic effects of sugar, and again, it shows that in the complete absence of the metabolic effects of sugar, highly palatable food that is high in reward value can drive increased consumption of calories and bodyweight gain.[189] The sweeteners themselves are calorie free, but just as with sugar, the increased palatability may make you *eat more total calories.*

For far too long, we have been stuck in Stone Age nutritional thought by trying to find the answers to what makes us fat in the inherent metabolic effects of specific nutrients. First it was, "It's fat that makes us fat. Let's all eat low-fat diets!" Then it was, "No, it's the carbs—the grains and the sugars and the insulin! Let's all eat low-carb!"

It's time for a paradigm shift.

The reason we're getting fatter isn't due to any specific macronutrient, and the solution to our predicament is not any diet based on jettisoning one or the other macronutrient from the diet.

Sugars and fats are ***not*** fattening due to their inherent metabolic properties—they're fattening when we consume them in highly rewarding processed foods, which act to drive up overall calorie consumption.

181 http://www.ncbi.nlm.nih.gov/pubmed/8140158

182 http://www.ncbi.nlm.nih.gov/pubmed/9023599

183 http://www.ncbi.nlm.nih.gov/pubmed/10336168

184 http://www.ncbi.nlm.nih.gov/pmc/articles/PMC2892765/

185 http://www.ncbi.nlm.nih.gov/pubmed/23088901

186 http://www.ncbi.nlm.nih.gov/pubmed/19634935

187 http://www.ncbi.nlm.nih.gov/pubmed/20060008

188 http://www.ncbi.nlm.nih.gov/pmc/articles/PMC2892765/

189 http://www.ncbi.nlm.nih.gov/pubmed/3200909

As Michael Moss explains, food is being willfully engineered to be addictive,[190] and there is simply no doubt that this is profoundly influencing the overall amount of calories we consume.

The key to understanding how food makes us fat is in food reward/palatability, not magical macronutrient ratios.

190 http://www.nytimes.com/2013/02/24/magazine/the-extraordinary-science-of-junk-food.html?pagewanted=all&_r=0

Fat vs. Sugar: Which is the Most Rewarding and Fattening?

So far, we've explained that neither sugar nor fat are fattening due to their inherent metabolic effects, but that *both can be fattening* when consumed in the form of highly palatable/rewarding processed foods.

The question that you're probably asking now is which of these nutrients does this more powerfully? Is it sugar or fat that stimulates increased calorie consumption and fat gain the most?

Well, one interesting study can give us an important clue in this regard. The study asked participants to replace a large portion of their normal daily intake of fat with either sugar or starch:

- **Group 1**: This group replaced 25% of their daily fat intake with simple carbohydrates (sugary foods)
- **Group 2**: This group replaced 25% of their daily fat intake with complex carbohydrates (both refined and unrefined starch foods)
- **Group 3**: This was the control group diet, which did not change their normal diet at all

All of these groups were eating *ad libitum* (according to their desire) and were not calorie controlled. This is important to see how much the palatability/reward of a particular type of diet drives up overall calorie consumption.

So what happened?

After 6 months on the various diets, the starch group (group 2) lost 9 pounds (4.25 kg), while the sugar group (group 1) and fat group (group 3) had no significant change. [191]

What does that mean?

It means that sugary and fatty foods are about equally as fattening, since replacing a large portion of fat with sugary foods did not cause any weight gain.

And it means that replacing fats with starchy carbohydrates actually tends to drive down food reward, thus decreasing overall calorie intake and causing weight loss. Therefore, starchy carbohydrates tend to be less fattening than either sugars or fats in the context of a typical diet

191 http://www.ncbi.nlm.nih.gov/pubmed/11756055

(again, not because of their inherent metabolic effects, but due to food reward factors affecting overall calories consumed).

This is, by the way, not the only study that has found this. Another similar (but shorter-term) study had very similar results—the high-starch diet decreased body fat much more than either the higher fat or high sucrose sugar diet.[192]

When we examine the reward value of different food groups, we see that added fats in the diet appear to be more rewarding than starch and about as rewarding as sugar (the very thing low-carb gurus demonize).[193]

So when you introduce added fats and oils into the diet, the combination of them being highly palatable, highly rewarding, having a high calorie density, and having fairly poor satiety relative to the calories they contain causes them to drive up overall calorie intake significantly without greatly increasing satiety. (Added refined fats do this in precisely the same way that added refined sugars do.) The end result of this is consuming more calories and getting as fat, or fatter, on higher-fat diets as compared to higher-carbohydrate diets.

The conclusion of all this is that carbohydrates and sugar are absolutely *not* uniquely fattening. Diets rich in carbohydrate or sugar **do not stimulate fat gain to a greater degree than diets where the majority of calories come from fats.**

In fact, the large increase in consumption of refined fats over the last century is—like refined sugars in processed foods—one of the reasons we consume more calories, and we're fatter now than we were 50 years ago.

One country—Australia—proves that quite clearly. **The Australian obesity epidemic has coincided with a significant increase in fat consumption and a *decrease* in sugar consumption!**[194 195]

---

192 http://www.ncbi.nlm.nih.gov/pubmed/9347402

193

194 http://www.ncbi.nlm.nih.gov/pmc/articles/PMC3257688/?tool=pubmed

195 Barclay, A., Brand-Miller, J. (2012). The Australian Paradox Revisited

Here are a couple of relevant quotes from the research:

> **"The findings confirm an 'Australian Paradox'—a substantial decline in refined sugars intake over the same timeframe that obesity has increased."**[196]

> "It is possible that less emphasis has been given to disseminating the message of lowering total energy intake, while avoidance of particular nutrients, such as sugars, has been the primary focus. ... Interestingly, research by WHO found **that the Australian energy supply has increased almost exclusively as a result of an increase in intake of fat**. ... Logic tells us that an inappropriately high intake of any energy source (alcohol, fat, protein, starch, or sugar) will result in weight gain. ... **Indeed, a literal interpretation of our findings would suggest that reductions in sugar intake may have contributed to the rise in obesity. Lowering the sugar content of foods may be counterproductive for weight management if there is replacement of sugars with refined or high glycemic index starches, saturated fats, or alcohol."**[197]

Thus, even if we were to say that it's not all carbs that make us fat, but specifically sugar that makes us fat (as if insulin secreted due to sugar is somehow different from insulin secreted due to other carbohydrates), we *still* cannot make a clear link between sugar consumption and obesity.

While sugar consumption did increase in the United States during the initial part of the obesity epidemic, it has actually been steadily *decreasing* over the last 15 years, while obesity rates continue to increase.[198]

Moreover, both the UK and Australian obesity epidemics have not only not occurred in conjunction with increased sugar consumption—they have occurred alongside a significant *decrease* in sugar consumption![199]

---

196 http://www.ncbi.nlm.nih.gov/pmc/articles/PMC3257688/?tool=pubmed

197 http://www.ncbi.nlm.nih.gov/pmc/articles/PMC3257688/?tool=pubmed

198 http://www.ncbi.nlm.nih.gov/pubmed/21753067

199 http://www.ncbi.nlm.nih.gov/pmc/articles/PMC3257688/?tool=pubmed

So this is clearly not a simple case of more sugar leads to more obesity.

Below you can see the trends in sugar consumption in the United States, UK, and Australia during the rise of obesity in those countries:

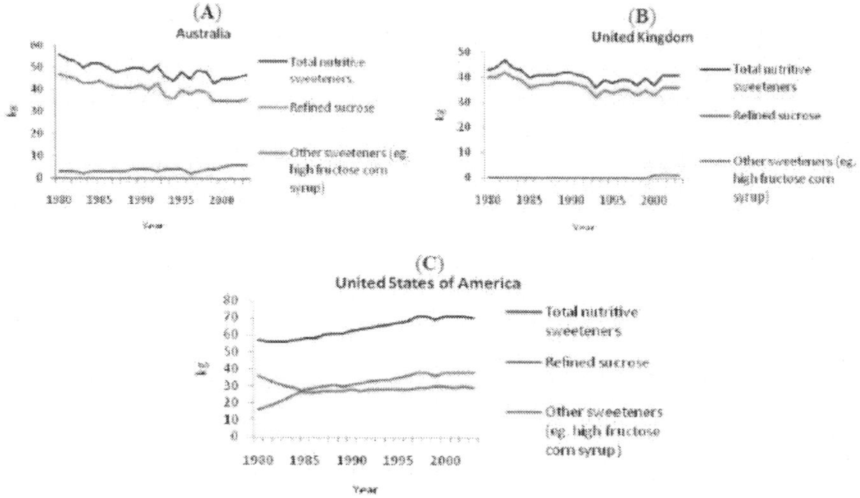

Here you can see the trend in sugar consumption in the United States, Australia, and the UK from 1980 to 2000. In the United States, sugar consumption has certainly increased, coinciding with the worsening of the American obesity epidemic. But in both the UK and Australia, sugar consumption actually decreased, coinciding with the worsening of their obesity epidemics.[200] *The fact that obesity epidemics can be dissociated from sugar consumption suggests that sugar consumption per se is definitely not THE cause of obesity.*

If sugar consumption is a cause of obesity, why is it that sugar consumption and obesity can be completely dissociated from one another—that you can have increasing obesity rates with *decreasing* intake of sugar?

The answer is that obesity epidemics are *not* driven by any one specific macronutrient or food group. They are driven by increased total *calorie* consumption.

200 http://www.mdpi.com/2072-6643/3/4/491

That increased calorie consumption, in turn, comes primarily from increased reward/palatability value of the diet—from processed foods rich in either sugars or fats (often both).

Moreover, these added sugars and fats are roughly equally potent stimulators of increased overall calorie intake.

Thus, if Americans had been given recommendations to eat a lower-carb, higher-fat diet (rather than a low-fat, higher-carbohydrate diet), and they had eaten a low-quality processed food diet that was high in fats and low in carbohydrates, we would be faced with the exact same obesity epidemic. And we already know this, since the Australian obesity epidemic confirms that obesity epidemics can coincide with decreased sugar consumption and increased fat consumption.

The simple reality is that if one is so inclined to myopic villainization of a specific macronutrient, it is possible to do so for either sugar or fat. As an example of how easy it would be to cherry-pick the evidence in either direction (to paint either sugar or fat as the primary cause of obesity), here is the conclusion of one meta-analysis that implicated sugar as being a significant cause of obesity:

> "Among free living people involving ad libitum diets, intake of free sugars or sugar sweetened beverages is a determinant of body weight. The change in body fatness that occurs with modifying intakes seems to be mediated via changes in energy intakes, since isoenergetic exchange of sugars with other carbohydrates was not associated with weight change." [201]

Here is another meta-analysis that implicated fat but not sugar:

> **"[A]lthough high intake of dietary fat is positively associated with indexes of obesity, high intake of sugar is negatively associated with indexes of obesity. There is ample reason to associate high-fat diets with obesity but, at present, no reason to associate high-sugar diets with obesity."[202]**

But again, overall the research does not strongly implicate either sugar or fat as being the major cause of fat gain. Obesity epidemics can occur (and have occurred) in conjunction with either an increase or

---

201 http://www.bmj.com/content/346/bmj.e7492

202 http://ajcn.nutrition.org/content/62/1/264S.abstract

decrease in sugar consumption and do not depend on the metabolic effects of any specific macronutrient. They depend on a food supply that is high in overall food reward/palatability, which can be driven by processed food products rich in either added sugars or added fats, since they drive up reward/palatability about equally as potently.

The proportion of carbohydrates to fat isn't the key factor here—the major nutritional factor driving obesity is highly rewarding/palatable processed foods.

A World Where Low-Carbers and Fruitarians are Both Lean!

So you might be wondering, "If high-fat diets are fattening, then why don't people on ultra-high-fat, low-carb diets not only not get fat, but often become leaner?"

Well, for the same reason that people who adopt fruitarian diets where they eat almost nothing but sugar also don't become fat and often become extremely lean!

The reason is that palatability and reward are actually quite low on *both* a diet of almost entirely fat and a diet of almost entirely fruit. When you are eating a diet of very limited food groups (and mostly whole foods), you actually tend not to eat very much food overall.

If you doubt that fruitarians eating a huge amount of sugar each day can be lean, I suggest browsing some fruitarian forums and letting some of the images of skinny fruitarians detonate in your brain.

But it's also an undebatable reality that people on extremely low-carb (or no-carb) and ultra-high-fat diets can be very lean.

Why? Simple. Such a diet is found to be extremely unpalatable by most people. Since ketogenic diets cause equal amounts of fat loss when controlled for calories, it is likely that the benefits many people claim to receive from ketogenic diets are not due to the magic of being a "fat burner" or "ketone burner" but simply due to how much they've lowered their overall calorie intake due to consuming a much lower reward/palatability diet. In fact, very low-carb and high-fat ketogenic diets are so incredibly unpalatable to most people that even when there is research indicating that a ketogenic diet is of proven medical benefit (such as in epilepsy), people have an incredibly hard time actually sticking to the diet due to its unpleasantness.[203] (We will explore this more in later chapters.)

The palatability sweet spot is where you have a diet that is already somewhat rich in carbs, and then you put a bunch of added fats into that diet. Or vice versa—you have a diet very rich in fatty foods, and then you add a bunch of sugar into the diet. That's when palatability rises off the charts and you really start chronically overconsuming calories. That's when you get an obesity epidemic. And that is precisely

203 http://www.ncbi.nlm.nih.gov/pubmed/7592151

what happened in the United States—we were eating a relatively high-fat diet and then added a bunch of refined grains and sugars on top of it (along with even *more fats)* to create a super-rewarding/palatable diet, and thus we started consuming hundreds of calories more each day. Other populations such as the Pima Indians did somewhat of the opposite—they started with a high-carb diet and added in tons of fat and became obese while eating a diet higher in fat and lower in carbs than they ate previously. The Australian obesity epidemic occurred in conjunction with decreased sugar intake and increased fat intake.

Adding lots of refined carbohydrates into a diet already high in fat tends to promote fat gain. So too does adding lots of refined fats into a carbohydrate-heavy diet.

In contrast, *unrefined* sugars and fats are not fattening, and if we had been given a recommendation to focus on purely unrefined whole foods—rather than a focus on carbohydrate vs. fat ratios—we would've likely halted the obesity epidemic far more effectively. (Assuming, of course, that people actually followed the advice, but that is another story altogether.)

One more time, so it really sinks in: The key factor that dictates whether food is fattening or not (i.e., how many total calories you consume) is *not* the inherent metabolic effects of any particular macronutrient or food group—it's due to the overall reward/palatability value of the diet.

This is why it is possible to be fat on either diets that are extremely high in fat (and low in carbs) or diets that are extremely high in sugar (but low in fat), and why it's possible to be lean on diets of those macronutrient compositions as well.

Do Whole Foods (or Bland Foods) Rich in Sugars Make You Fat or Lean?

We just explained that there is nothing inherently fattening about the metabolic effects of sugar, and that any fattening effect that does occur is primarily a result of sweet tastes driving up overall calorie consumption.

So the natural question then is what happens when sugar is consumed in large amounts in foods that don't taste especially delicious? (This could be foods intentionally designed not to taste particularly sweet, or simple whole foods rich in sugar, like fruit.)

Here's where things get really interesting because, all of the sudden, a high-sugar diet can now lead to remarkable amounts of fat *loss*!

- A study by Madero et al. compared effects of calorie-matched diets that were either low-fructose (less than 20 g/day) or moderate-fructose (50-70 g/day) mostly from whole fruit on overweight people for 6 weeks. What did they find? The moderate-fructose group lost significantly more weight than the low-fructose group (4.19 kg versus 2.83 kg, respectively). The authors concluded, "For weight loss achievement, an energy-restricted moderate natural fructose diet was superior to a low-fructose diet."[204]
- A 1971 paper titled "Physiological Effects of a Mainly Fruit Diet in Man" had subjects eat nothing but fruit (82% of kcal) and nuts (18% of kcal) for six months while eating however much food they wanted. The diet was a very low protein (5.6-8%), moderate fat (37-45%), and high-carbohydrate diet (52-65%). In other words, these people consumed the majority of their daily calories in the form of unrefined sugar for 6 months. What was the result? Their body weights approached the "theoretical ideal," with lean subjects remaining lean and overweight subjects losing large amounts of body fat. [205] This study very clearly shows that sugar is *not* inherently fattening, and when the sugar is consumed in the form of low- to moderate-reward foods, it can actually promote fat *loss*.

---

204 http://www.ncbi.nlm.nih.gov/pubmed/21621801

205 http://www.ncbi.nlm.nih.gov/pubmed/4928686

- A meta-analysis that examined the relationship between fruit intake and body weight found this: "We identified three intervention, eight prospective observational, and five cross-sectional studies that explored this relationship. **Two of the intervention studies showed that fruit intake reduced body weight, five of the prospective observational studies showed that fruit consumption reduced the risk of developing overweight and obesity, and four of the cross-sectional studies found an inverse association between fruit intake and body weight. ... [T]he majority of the evidence points towards a possible inverse association between fruit intake and overweight."**[206]
- Perhaps the most dramatic study showing the effects of consuming a high-sugar diet that is low in food reward/palatability is a 1965 study that involved feeding subjects a bland liquid diet through a dispensing straw.[207] In the study, which involved both lean and obese volunteers, participants were given a very simple instruction: to eat no other food than the liquid food, but to eat as much of the liquid food as they wanted, whenever they pleased. The result? **Lean volunteers ate a normal amount of calories and maintained weight, but obese volunteers dramatically and spontaneously reduced their caloric intake and lost fat rapidly—doing so *without* any hunger. One obese man lost 200 pounds in 255 days without hunger.** As Guyenet notes, "This is exactly what one would expect if unpalatable/unrewarding food lowered the biologically 'defended' level of fat mass. Interestingly, the diet was high in sugar but was otherwise very low in palatability/reward value."[208] Other studies have confirmed these findings.[209]

---

206 http://onlinelibrary.wiley.com/doi/10.1111/j.1467-789X.2009.00582.x/abstract?deniedAccessCustomisedMessage=&userIsAuthenticated=false

207 http://www.ncbi.nlm.nih.gov/pubmed/5216999

208 http://wholehealthsource.blogspot.com/2011/10/case-for-food-reward-hypothesis-of_07.html

209 http://www.ncbi.nlm.nih.gov/pubmed/1013218

There is nothing inherently fattening about sugar.

When sugar is consumed in a way that is not particularly tasty (at least not *unnaturally* tasty), it not only does not cause increased consumption of overall calories, it can actually dramatically *lower* calorie intake and cause fat *loss*—to the extent that when overweight and obese people replace processed foods in their diet in favor of natural fruit sugars (or other relatively bland sugar-rich foods), they reliably lose fat and approach their ideal weights.

What dictates whether a food is fattening or not is *not* a question of fat vs carbs/sugar. It isn't even the type of fat or sugar. This does not have much if anything to do with questions of saturated versus unsaturated, polyunsaturated versus monounsaturated. This doesn't have to do with high-glycemic-index carbs versus low-glycemic-index carbs, or sugars versus starches, or glucose versus fructose. The answer to whether a food is fattening or not is *not found in any of those things (or any combination of them)!* **Thus, looking for the answers to the question of what makes us fat from the framework of trying to blame it on some specific macronutrient or specific type of a single macronutrient is fundamentally misguided.** At best, the effects from any of these factors are relatively minor.

What dictates whether a food is fattening is primarily reward and palatability.

When you consume a diet rich in fats from whole foods, they are generally conducive to slimming rather than fattening. When you consume a diet rich in fats in the form of added fats in processed foods, they will generally be fattening.

The same goes for sugars—added sugars will generally be fattening, while a diet composed largely of whole-food sugars will generally be slimming.

The magic isn't in the specific nutrients themselves—it's all in the packaging.

When you consume sugars in the form of whole foods, they are clearly not fattening in any way. And if one is overweight, the evidence indicates that eating a high-sugar diet that is from whole foods (or bland liquids) frequently results in remarkable amounts of fat loss.

When Food Really Does Make Us Fat: Conclusions

So how can we make sense of everything we've looked at so far, which shows that the obesity epidemic can't be blamed on one specific macronutrient?

One interesting study sought to do just that: It's called "The Real Contribution of Added Sugars and Fats to Obesity."

To pull out a few highlights from the abstract:

"Obesity rates in the United States are a function of socioeconomic status. Higher rates are found among groups with lower educational and income levels, among racial and ethnic minorities, and in high-poverty areas. Yet, the relation between obesity, nutrition, and diet continues to be viewed in biologic terms, with the search for likely causes focused on consumption of specific macronutrients, foods, or food groups. … Plausible physiologic mechanisms have included the metabolic effects of dietary components, mostly sugars and fats, on regulation of food intake and deposition of body fat. **However, the evidence could not have been convincing since the blame for rising obesity rates seems to shift regularly, every 10 years or so, from fats to sugars and then back again.**

"This review demonstrates that much of past epidemiologic research is consistent with a single parsimonious explanation: obesity has been linked repeatedly to consumption of low-cost foods.

"Refined grains, added sugars, and added fats are inexpensive, good tasting, and convenient. In other words, the low cost of dietary energy (dollars/megajoule), rather than specific food, beverage, or macronutrient choices, may be the main predictor of population weight gain."[210]

This study gets one very important thing right: the researchers see the big picture that the evidence does not show that *any* specific macronutrient or food group (i.e., fats, carbs, sugars) can be singled out as being *the cause* (or a major cause) of fat gain.

It rightly points out that the search for good solutions to fat loss does *not* rest in the extent to which one eats "low-fat" or "low-carb" and that the evidence is obviously not convincing since public opinion

---

210 http://www.ncbi.nlm.nih.gov/pubmed/17591599

and health gurus routinely shift from demonizing fat to carbs to fat and back to carbs again.

For that reason, this study is superior to countless studies conducted by researchers that are searching for answers by trying to blame fat gain on one specific food group or another.

The study also correctly points out that low-cost processed food—rather than a specific macronutrient like sugar or fat—is what is really linked with obesity. The problem with this study is that it tries to create a parsimonious explanation for this link solely through the framework of food costs.

While food costs are undoubtedly partially at play, the bigger factor at play here is that low-cost processed foods are extremely calorie dense and highly rewarding/palatable and thus drive up overall calorie consumption tremendously (while also disrupting the brain's ability to regulate energy balance).[211] [212] [213]

So a better explanation to all the conflicting data that singles out either fats or sugars as being "the cause" is this: the low cost of processed food and, to a greater extent, the *higher palatability/reward* value of such foods causes us to consume more overall calories and thus drives fat gain.

There are, of course, several other factors at play with regard to how food (or eating habits) can make us fat:

- High food variety
- High calorie density of foods (and high calorie to satiety ratio) and passive overconsumption
- Low cost of food per calorie
- Low need for physical effort to acquire or consume food (no hunting or gathering or cultivation needed)
- Eating for entertainment rather than physical hunger
- Eating for pleasure rather than physical hunger
- Eating for socialization rather than physical hunger
- Eating out of habit rather than physical hunger

---

211 http://www.foodandnutritionresearch.net/index.php/fnr/article/view/5144/5755

212 http://www.sciencedirect.com/science/article/pii/S0031938404001842

213 http://jn.nutrition.org/content/133/3/831S.full

- Eating to soothe oneself emotionally rather than to satiate physical hunger

All of these factors can significantly increase total calorie intake and drive fat gain.

It is also important to remember that food is just one of several factors at play with regard to the obesity epidemic. Other factors such as circadian rhythm, exercise, stress, genetics, developmental factors, and NEAT (non-exercise activity thermogenesis) all have important roles to play as well. So one should keep that bigger picture in mind in any discussion of what nutritional factors are fattening or not.

But in terms of how the food itself contributes to fat gain, it is likely that reward/palatability of food is the major player.

In the words of Guyenet:

> **"[T]he more I read, the more I'm convinced that excessive food reward and/or palatability is the elephant in the room when it comes to obesity and metabolic dysfunction. We live our lives surrounded by foods that are professionally crafted to satisfy our basest gustatory desires—to drive us to eat more, against the wisdom that our bodies have accumulated over millions of years. They do this by exploiting the hard-wired preferences that guided us towards healthy food in the natural environment."** [214]

What makes us fat isn't any specific macronutrient or subtype of macronutrient.

Fattening foods are foods of any macronutrient ratio—whether high in carbs or low in carbs, high in sugar or low in sugar, low in fat or high in fat—which are *unnaturally* rewarding/highly palatable and thus drive up *overall calorie consumption.*

214 http://wholehealthsource.blogspot.com/2011/06/food-reward-dominant-factor-in-obesity_28.html

SUMMARY

- **What dictates whether a food is fattening or not is not the inherent metabolic and hormonal effects of a particular nutrient like sugar or fat.**
- **The primary factor that dictates whether a dietary pattern is fattening or not is food reward/palatability and how that influences the overall number of calories that are consumed.** Other important factors include high food variety, high calorie to satiety ratio, low cost of food per calorie, low need for physical effort to acquire food, overall abundance and ease of accessibility of high variety of highly rewarding foods with a high calorie to satiety ratio that can be consumed with minimal calorie expenditure. These are the major dietary factors that influence net caloric balance. The research does not indicate that any macronutrient—either fat or sugar—is particularly responsible for fat gain or is necessary to jettison from one's diet in order to lose fat. Overall, caloric balance is what determines body composition, not the ratio of carbs to fats in the diet.
    - Thus anyone who is speaking about how food makes us fat through the lens of the inherent metabolic effects of certain macronutrients—for instance, trying to blame either carbs/sugars or fats as being the major thing causing us to be fat (e.g., "fat makes you fat" or "sugar makes you fat" or "carbs boost insulin, which is a fat-storing hormone")—is fundamentally wrong and deeply misguided.
- **In terms of food reward/palatability, fats drive up overall calorie consumption at least as much as, or more than, carbohydrates do. Refined fats and refined sugars are roughly equal in terms of how much they increase overall calories consumed, and thus how fattening they are.**
- Sugar, including fructose, is not inherently fattening relative to other calorie sources. **And, even in non-calorie restricted diets (ad libitum), unrefined sugar consumption is compatible with fat loss in the context of simple whole-food diets.**

- **Sugar can be fattening in certain contexts, specifically if it is added to foods and beverages in a way that increases their palatability, reward value, and calorie to satiety ratio. Note that this is precisely the same context in which fat becomes fattening.**
- **Refined sugars and fats are roughly equally fattening.** The notion that "fat doesn't make you fat—sugar does" is fundamentally false. In reality, refined fats and sugars drive up calorie intake and fatten us up about equally well.
- If the goal is fat loss, the solution is *not* in any specific fat versus carbohydrate ratio, or in the inherent metabolic/hormonal effects of carbs versus fat. **It is much wiser to focus on *where* the fats and carbohydrates in your diet are coming from and what level of reward/palatability they have—that is, whether they are consumed in the form of added refined sugars or fats that are in processed food products, or in the form of lower reward/palatability fats and sugars as in whole foods. This is likely the single most important factor that dictates whether your diet is fattening or not.**
- Sugar-sweetened beverages are probably one of the most fattening elements of the modern diet. This effect is likely driven by a combination of altered calorie to satiety ratio of consuming large amounts of calories in liquid form and due to reward/palatability factors.
- **Sugar in whole food form—from fruit—is not fattening. If anything, it's slimming.**

<u>Here are the practical take-home messages for those who want to lose fat:</u>

- **Avoid processed foods that have large amounts of added refined sugars and/or fats. Avoid adding large amounts of purified sugars or fats to your meals.**
- **Avoid sugar-sweetened beverages** (soda, punch, coffee with added sugars and fats, possibly fruit juice, cocktails, etc.).
- **Eat your fruit!** Do not fear whole-food sugars. Sugars in the form of whole foods contain a low calorie to satiety ratio and a moderate palatability and reward value. Eating fruit does not

contribute to fat gain, and if anything, consuming a whole-food diet with ample fruit is likely to contribute to leanness.

Following these principles is likely to prevent fat gain and, to the extent that one is currently engaging in consuming foods with large amounts of added sugars and/or fats, will induce fat loss.

Chapter 4: Debunking the Myth that Carbohydrates/Sugars Cause Insulin Resistance and Type II Diabetes

The basic idea of the low-carb gurus is that eating carbs "spikes" blood sugar levels, which causes a rise in the "evil, fat-storing, diabetes-causing hormone" insulin. Because type II diabetes is often over-simplistically thought by many people to be a problem of "too much blood sugar" or "too much insulin," it appears on the surface that carbohydrates must be the obvious culprit, given that carbohydrates do indeed spike blood sugar and insulin levels.

The basic line of thinking is, "Carbs spike blood sugar levels and insulin levels, and if you do that frequently, those transient blood sugar/insulin spikes turn into a chronic excess of blood sugar and insulin." And that's how we get insulin resistance and type II diabetes, according to the low-carb gurus.

Here is Gary Taubes saying the same thing:

> **"Anything that increases insulin, induces insulin resistance, and induces the pancreas to compensate by secreting still more insulin, will also lead to an excess accumulation of body fat."** [215]

215 Taubes, G. Good Calories, Bad Calories

Here is Mark Hyman, MD talking about what insulin resistance is, and what causes it, in his book, *UltraMetabolism:*

> **"Insulin resistance is a condition where you develop a tolerance to insulin and produce excess amounts of insulin. Generally this is because you eat too many sugars or bad carbs."[216]**

As we're about to find out, this conceptualization of what insulin resistance is and what causes it is a bunch of pseudoscientific nonsense. Insulin resistance is not caused by insulin itself or by carbohydrates--not even sugars and "bad carbs." It is actually rather remarkable how this idea that carbohydrates cause diabetes—which has no real basis in science—has found its way into popular culture so much so that not only do regular average lay people now think it's true, but even some popular health guru MDs are promulgating this pseudoscience.

The notion that carbohydrates cause insulin resistance and type II diabetes is one of the biggest myths that we have in the nutrition realm today (along with the myth that dietary cholesterol is the cause of heart disease). This myth—which has been fervently promoted by low-carb gurus—basically asserts that the more you eat carbs, raise blood sugar, and stimulate insulin, the more the insulin mechanism "wears out." Then, boom! Before you know it, diabetes! (Interesting how low-carb gurus adamantly refute the myth that eating saturated fat/cholesterol causes heart disease while simultaneously perpetuating another equally harmful myth—that eating carbs causes diabetes.)

It is actually a very logical theory that appears to make sense on the surface. Just like it makes logical sense that eating cholesterol is what causes cholesterol plaques to accumulate on your artery walls, it also makes sense that eating things that boost blood sugar and insulin would be the cause of perpetually high levels of insulin and high blood sugar. Since diabetes is characterized by an excess of blood sugar, it is easy to speculate that diabetes would be simply the result of taking in too many carbs. After all, carbs turn to sugar in your blood, and diabetes is a disease of too much sugar in the blood, so what could possibly be wrong with that logic?

While that logic does seem to make sense on the surface (which is probably why nearly everyone believes it), it has essentially no basis in

---

216 Hyamn, M. Ultrametabolism

science. In fact, as we're about to show you, there is no significant scientific evidence showing that consuming carbohydrates—even high-glycemic carbohydrates—causes insulin resistance and type II diabetes.

So, let's address this claim systematically, in the spirit of science. The claim that carbohydrates cause insulin resistance/type II diabetes can be tested rather easily in several direct and indirect ways:

- Look at studies where they examine groups of people who eat more carbohydrates/sugars versus other groups of people, and check whether those consuming more carbohydrates actually do have higher rates of insulin resistance/type II diabetes, as the carbs-cause-diabetes theory would predict.
- Examine cultures that are undergoing a diabetes epidemic and check to see if that diabetes epidemic is paralleled by increased carbohydrate consumption.
- Examine randomized controlled studies where they give high-carb or high-sugar diets to one group and lower carb/sugar intake to another group, and see if the higher carb/sugar intakes cause insulin resistance/type II diabetes.

Any one of these would likely give us the answer to this question, but for the sake of thoroughness, let's examine all three. Let's start with #1.

Does Eating Carbohydrates Cause Insulin Resistance?

First things first. It shouldn't be too hard to figure out if eating carbs is the cause of insulin resistance and diabetes—all we have to do is look at groups of people around the world eating totally different amounts of carbs and sugars, and see if the ones eating lots of carbs/sugars have higher rates of insulin resistance/diabetes than populations eating fewer carbohydrates/sugars.

If we look around the world to find the populations eating the most carbohydrates, we find groups like the Okinawans, Kitavans, the Tukisenta of Papua New Guinea, and the Ewe tribe in West Africa. These populations all eat radically more of their daily calories from carbohydrates than those of us in the United States, where we eat about 50% of our daily calories from carbohydrates. So let's see if they have diabetes:

The Kitavans: Dr. Staffan Lindeberg researched this population heavily during the 1990s and found that their diet consisted mostly of taro, sweet potatoes, cassava, fruit, coconut, and seafood. They ate about 50g a day of unrefined sugar from fruit. Their diet came in at 69% carbohydrate—again, much higher than in the United States. Lindeberg found that there were literally no cases of overweight or diabetes on the entire island! Their fasting insulin level (a measure of insulin resistance and diabetes) was extremely low, and diabetes and heart disease were unheard of on the island. [217]

The Kuna of Panama: 65% carbohydrate diet (with some refined sugar, doughnuts, and Kool-Aid) and still no incidence of type II diabetes.[218]

The Okinawans: They eat a diet made up of a whopping 85% carbohydrates (9% protein, 6% fat), mainly from starchy sweet potatoes, and had minimal incidence of diabetes prior to Westernization.[219]

---

217 http://wholehealthsource.blogspot.com/2008/08/kitavans-wisdom-from-pacific-islands.html

218 http://wholehealthsource.blogspot.com/2008/03/say-hello-to-kuna.html

219 http://chriskresser.com/is-starch-a-beneficial-nutrient-or-a-toxin

The Tukisenta of Papua New Guinea: They eat a diet of over 90% carbohydrates and have been documented as having no incidences of type II diabetes.[220]

The Hadza of Tanzania: This population eats a diet of mostly carbohydrates. They get their carbohydrate from starchy tubers and consume a large portion of it from sugar-rich foods like honey, baobab fruit, and berries.[221] They have virtually no type II diabetes or insulin resistance.

The Tarahumara Indians of Mexico: This group—who is related to the Pima Indians, who have the highest rates of diabetes in the world while eating a high-fat diet—eats a traditional diet of mostly corn, beans, rice, and squash, and has an extremely low incidence of type II diabetes. Their diet is 12% fat and over 75% carbohydrate.[222]

The Ewe Tribe in West Africa: This population eats a diet of essentially nothing but starchy tubers. The diet is up to 84% carbohydrate by some estimates.[223] They have excellent insulin sensitivity and no incidence of type II diabetes.

If eating carbohydrates is the cause of insulin resistance/type II diabetes, how is it that numerous populations around the world who eat far more carbohydrates than the paltry 50% of daily calories that Americans eat have dramatically *lower* incidences of type II diabetes? How is it that populations that eat almost nothing but insulin-spiking carbohydrates all day, every day for six or seven decades have negligible to nonexistent rates of type II diabetes? This simple fact is our first clue that insulin resistance is *not* simply a matter of eating carbs (or things that spike insulin).

We can also do studies that directly check for a link between carbohydrate consumption and insulin resistance. In fact, these experiments have been done extensively, and they virtually never find a link between carbohydrate consumption and insulin resistance:

---

220 http://wholehealthsource.blogspot.com/2011/08/carbohydrate-hypothesis-of-obesity.html

221 http://wholehealthsource.blogspot.com/2012/06/sugar-intake-and-body-fatness-in-non.html

222 http://ajcn.nutrition.org/content/32/4/905.full.pdf

223 http://www.weightymatters.ca/2012/09/the-ewe-super-high-carb-diet-992.html

- "Total carbohydrate, dietary fiber, fruit fiber, vegetable fiber, legume fiber, glycemic load, and refined grain intakes were not associated with prevalence of the metabolic syndrome." [224]
- "Habitual intake of diets ... with a high content of total carbohydrate including simple sugars was not associated with the probability of having insulin resistance." [225]
- "The available data support the idea that consumption of diets high in total carbohydrate does not adversely affect insulin sensitivity compared with high-fat diets."[226]
- The latest meta-analysis (data compiled from a comprehensive review of the scientific studies) on the subject published in 2014 found *no* benefit on insulin sensitivity in overweight people from carbohydrate restriction—even among those with type II diabetes: "There is probably little or no difference in weight loss and changes in cardiovascular risk factors up to two years of follow-up when overweight and obese adults, with or without type 2 diabetes, are randomized to low CHO (low-carb) diets and isoenergetic balance (higher-carb diets that are equal in calories)." [227]

Obviously, if it were simply "things that spike insulin" (i.e., carbohydrates) that are *the* cause of insulin resistance, there would be a very clear and obvious correlation between carbohydrate consumption and insulin resistance in all of these studies. It would be very easy to notice such a phenomenon, and hundreds of studies would've proven this by now. Yet, the science shows no such link.

---

224 http://www.ncbi.nlm.nih.gov/pubmed/14747241

225 http://www.ncbi.nlm.nih.gov/pubmed/15920058

226 http://www.ncbi.nlm.nih.gov/pubmed/11584106

227 (http://www.plosone.org/article/info%3Adoi%2F10.1371%2Fjournal.pone.0100652)

In Cultures Undergoing a Diabetes Epidemic, is That Skyrocketing of Diabetes Incidence Paralleled by Increased Carbohydrate Consumption?

First, let's look at the most famous population that has undergone a diabetes epidemic—the Pima Indians, who are, in fact, the most diabetic population on the planet. During the span of time that they have gone from having negligible rates of diabetes to being the most diabetic group on Earth, we should expect to see an increase in carbohydrate consumption, right?

Here's what we actually see:

The traditional Pima diet was a high-carbohydrate diet consisting of beans, corn, and squash, with wild fish, game meat, and plants. *"Researchers at the NIDDK in Phoenix have estimated that the traditional Pima diet took about 70 percent of its calories in the form of carbohydrates, 15 percent in protein, and 15 percent in fat. By the 1950s the proportions had changed to 61 percent carbohydrate, 15 percent in protein, and 24 percent in fat.* ***In 1971 it was 44 percent carbohydrate, 12 percent protein, and 44 percent fat–a tripling of the fat content."***[228]

If carbohydrate is the cause of insulin resistance, it's rather peculiar that the most diabetic population on Earth became diabetic in conjunction with a massive decrease in carbohydrate consumption and an increase in fat consumption.

Always worth noting is that the US Pimas—eating a processed food diet—have the highest rate of diabetes in the world (38%), while the Mexican Pimas—who still eat their traditional high-carbohydrate diet—have a rate of diabetes under 6.9%.

What if we look at the United States as a whole—a country that has recently undergone an obesity epidemic? Over the last century, the incidence of type II diabetes has skyrocketed in the United States. This is an undeniable fact. Now, if carbohydrates are the cause of insulin resistance/type II diabetes, we should, of course, see that an increased intake of carbohydrates parallels this diabetes epidemic. Right? Just as we *do* see an increase in calorie consumption paralleling the diabetes epidemic—thus clearly showing that increased *calorie* consumption parallels diabetes—if carbohydrates cause insulin resistance/diabetes,

---

228 Campos, P. The Obesity Myth.

then carbohydrate consumption should have also gone up in parallel to the increase in diabetes.

If we take a short view of just the last three or four decades, carbohydrate consumption has gone up to some extent. However, if we take the long view over the last 100 years, carbohydrate consumption has not changed significantly! Carbohydrate consumption has actually *not* gone up—100 years ago, it was around 50% of our daily calories, and now it's roughly the same. The only thing that has increased significantly over that time is fat intake.[229]

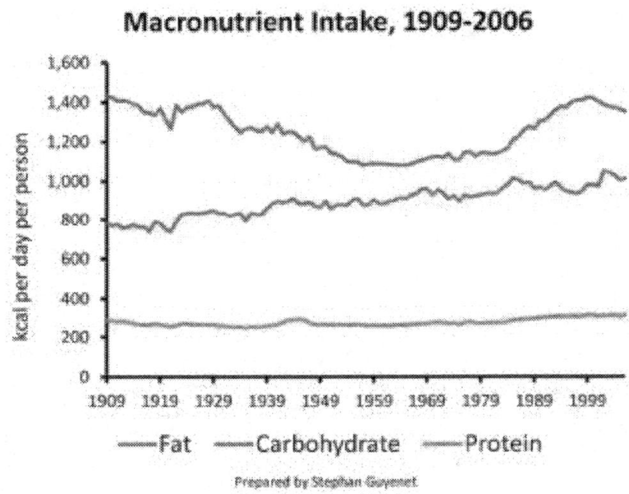

(Source: Guyenet, S. *The Carbohydrate Hypothesis of Obesity - a Critical Examination)*

How can carbohydrate consumption be causing the diabetes epidemic when carbohydrate consumption clearly does not parallel the diabetes epidemic?

During the epidemic of obesity and diabetes in Australia, the only macronutrient that has increased significantly is dietary fat. [230] [231]

If we can see diabetes epidemics occurring without any increase in carbohydrate consumption—even a huge *decrease* in carbohydrate

229 http://wholehealthsource.blogspot.com/2011/08/carbohydrate-hypothesis-of-obesity.html

230 http://www.ncbi.nlm.nih.gov/pmc/articles/PMC3257688/?tool=pubmed

231 Barclay, A., Brand-Miller, J. (2012). The Australian Paradox Revisited

consumption (as was the case with the Pima Indians)—this clearly shows us that carbohydrates are not causing diabetes.

But wait! There is still one hole in the above logic—we didn't distinguish between different types of carbohydrates. Maybe carbohydrates in general do not cause insulin resistance, but maybe sugars, refined carbohydrates, and the so-called "bad carbs" do.

Are High-Glycemic, Sugary Carbs Causing Diabetes?"

Now, if you're really up on the history of nutrient consumption in the United States, you would know that even though carbohydrate consumption hasn't gone up over the last 100 years (as we just explained), consumption of high-glycemic carbs (i.e., sugars) has gone up over that time.

So maybe you think, "Oh, well maybe carbs aren't the cause of diabetes, but high-glycemic (GI), insulin-spiking carb sources are?"

It's a valid thought, since high GI carbohydrate consumption has clearly increased over the last century. So let's see if any studies have tested this simple idea. Sure enough, there are numerous studies that have tested this hypothesis.

Strangely enough, the majority of these studies find no significant relationship between glycemic index of the diet (i.e., eating lots of sugary carbs) versus eating a low-glycemic-index diet (i.e., few or no sugary carbs) and insulin resistance. For as many studies as one can find that appear to implicate sugar as being correlated with insulin resistance (such as this one or this one), there are as many or more showing either no correlation or an inverse correlation. Some studies have even shown *higher* fasting insulin (i.e., more insulin resistance) on the *low-glycemic-index diet.*

Lau et al. noted, "Habitual intake of diets with a high glycemic index and high glycemic load or diets with a high content of total carbohydrate including simple sugars was not associated with the probability of having insulin resistance."[232]

Several studies have actually found significant inverse associations between sugar intake and type II diabetes—that is, those who consumed more sugar had *less* of an incidence of type II diabetes.[233] [234]

According to research published in the journal *Diabetes Care*, "Prevailing beliefs over the past 20 years regarding sugars and diabetes admonished that added sugar, primarily sucrose, should be avoided

---

232 http://www.ncbi.nlm.nih.gov/pubmed/15920058

233 http://nutrigen.ph.ucla.edu/files/view/pubs/03sugar-diabetes.pdf

234 Meyer KA, Kushi LH, Jacobs DR Jr, Slavin J, Sellers TA, Folsom AR: Carbohydrates, dietary fiber, and incident type 2 diabetes in older women. Am J Clin Nutr 71:921–930, 2000

and that naturally occurring sugars should be restricted in the diabetic diet. Support for these beliefs was based largely on results from animal and human studies suggesting that simple sugars would confer a higher postprandial glycemia than starch. Consequently, diets for diabetic patients have been sugar restricted for fear of stimulating hyperglycemia, exaggerating insulin response to carbohydrates, and causing possible cardiomyocyte dysfunction, and/or accelerated loss of β-cells. However, **several metabolic studies have reported that inclusion of a moderate amount of dietary sucrose within a balanced diabetic diet did not elicit subsequent deleterious effects on glycemic control."** [235]

The simple fact is this: While there are some observational studies linking GI and insulin resistance, numerous well-controlled studies—some over a year long--have shown that glycemic index simply does not have a significant impact on either insulin sensitivity or body fatness.[236] [237] [238] [239]

In perhaps one of the most significant studies done on the subject, done for 6 months with 720 participants (one of the longest and largest studies ever on the subject), participants were assigned to eat either a diet of:

- High saturated fat, high glycemic index
- High monounsaturated fat, high glycemic index
- High monounsaturated fat, low glycemic index
- Low fat, high glycemic index
- Low fat, low glycemic index

Naturally, researchers expected that the first group—those eating a diet high in both saturated fat and high-glycemic carbs—would have

235 http://care.diabetesjournals.org/content/26/4/1008.long

236 http://wholehealthsource.blogspot.com/2010/08/saturated-fat-glycemic-index-and.html

237 http://wholehealthsource.blogspot.com/2009/03/its-time-to-let-go-of-glycemic-index.html

238 http://wholehealthsource.blogspot.com/2009/03/more-thoughts-on-glycemic-index.html

239 http://www.ncbi.nlm.nih.gov/pubmed/14747241

the worst insulin sensitivity. Yet, after 6 months, there were no detectable differences in insulin sensitivity between the groups. [240]

> Other researchers analyzed dozens of studies conducted on the subject and concluded, "In our large cohort of 38,480 initially healthy postmenopausal women followed for an average of 6 years, we accrued 918 incident cases of type 2 diabetes and found no definitive influence of sugar intake on the risk of developing type 2 diabetes. ... **Sucrose intake was inversely associated with the risk of type 2 diabetes with marginal significance (P = 0.05), whereas fructose, glucose, and lactose did not appear to be significantly associated with the risk of type 2 diabetes."** [241]

Guyenet concluded his review of the research on this topic by noting, "Overall, these studies do not support the idea that lowering the glycemic index of carbohydrate foods is useful for weight loss, insulin or glucose control, or anything else besides complicating your life."[242]

If sugar (or high glycemic index carbohydrates) were a major cause—let alone *the* cause—of insulin resistance and type II diabetes, dozens of studies would show an enormous and very obvious correlation between the two. This would be an incredibly easy thing to prove.

Yet numerous studies either show very small positive correlations, no correlation at all, or even inverse correlations!

What these studies make abundantly clear is that sugar consumption is not a significant cause of insulin resistance/type II diabetes.

If sugar's inherent metabolic effects are causal of insulin resistance at all, the effect is so miniscule that dozens of studies deliberately trying to look for an effect are not able to detect any relationship whatsoever.

The science is very clear on the subject—neither carbs nor sugar are the cause of insulin resistance and type II diabetes.

---

240 http://ajcn.nutrition.org/content/early/2010/08/25/ajcn.2009.29096.abstract

241 http://nutrigen.ph.ucla.edu/files/view/pubs/03sugar-diabetes.pdf

242 http://wholehealthsource.blogspot.com/2009/03/its-time-to-let-go-of-glycemic-index.html

Fructose, and How It Compares to the Insulin Resistance-Inducing Effects of a High-Fat Diet

The only type of carbohydrate that one can find even a shred of a link to insulin resistance to is fructose. And interestingly, fructose causes the smallest increase in insulin of just about any sugar—it's actually the *lowest glycemic index* of all natural sugars with a very low glycemic index of just 19—so even this doesn't support Taubes' hypothesis that anything that boosts insulin transiently is the cause of insulin resistance.

Recently, studies have found that extremely high intakes of fructose can induce insulin resistance—though this typically requires consumption of *pure* fructose (which is virtually never consumed by humans, since we don't eat foods that contain only fructose by itself) in amounts well beyond what could be achieved on any normal human diet. According to Guyenet, "In humans, high-dose refined fructose feeding can cause insulin resistance in as little as a week, however this requires an amount of fructose that far exceeds what can be obtained in a normal diet. Somewhat lower, but still very high (~100 g/d) fructose intakes do not lead to insulin resistance in healthy, lean adults when fed for four weeks."[243]

In addition, it's worth pointing out that the evidence is far from conclusive in pointing to fructose as a significant cause of insulin resistance, considering that there are some studies that show profound *benefits* of fructose consumption on health markers related to insulin resistance. [244] [245]

Even with high doses of refined fructose, the link with insulin resistance is weak. For contrast, it's worth noting that if one was looking to cherry-pick evidence to blame insulin resistance on specific

243 http://wholehealthsource.blogspot.com/2012/01/what-causes-insulin-resistance-part-v.html

244 http://www.ncbi.nlm.nih.gov/pubmed/22354959

245 http://suppversity.blogspot.com/2012/08/6x-bananas-day-meta-analysis-lower.html

nutrients, one can find numerous studies showing that insulin resistance can be induced quite easily on a high-fat diet.[246] [247] [248]

This is particularly interesting considering that low-carb diet advocates often villainize carbs/sugar/fructose and espouse eating a low-carb, high-fat diet, explicitly for the reason that it would be better to protect against insulin resistance/diabetes. This is an assertion built on the notion that carbs cause insulin resistance and fats do not, which is patently false.

One interesting rodent study compared the effects of eating a high-fructose diet (something low-carb advocates claim will make you diabetic and obese) versus eating a high-fat diet (which is commonly advocated by low-carb gurus):

"The 10-week high-fat diet led to obesity and low IS [low IS = high insulin resistance], whereas rats fed with the high-fructose diet exhibited no change in IS [insulin resistance] and lipidaemia. The high-fat diet had more deleterious response than high-fructose diet to induce obesity and low IS in rats."[249]

Interestingly, the first study to address the question of how diets that vary in carbohydrate and fat content affect insulin resistance was published in 1935 by Dr. H.P. Himsworth. He found that not only do very high carbohydrate intakes *not* cause insulin resistance, they actually do the opposite! He found that insulin sensitivity was increased by feeding a high-carbohydrate diet and decreased by feeding a very *low*-carbohydrate diet. This was particularly true in the extremes—that is, extremely high carbohydrate intakes enhanced insulin sensitivity, and extremely low-carbohydrate intakes decreased it. (This is largely an adaptive insulin resistance. Because the brain's major source of fuel is glucose, when glucose/carbohydrate intake is low in the diet, the body's cells desensitize to insulin in order to spare what little carbohydrate is present in the diet for the body's most vital organ—the brain.)

However, in addition to this sort of adaptive insulin resistance that we see on ultra-low-carbohydrate diets, very high-fat diets have been

---

246 http://www.ncbi.nlm.nih.gov/pubmed/15297079

247 http://classic.ajpendo.physiology.org/content/251/5/E576.short

248 http://www.ncbi.nlm.nih.gov/pubmed/12643169

249 http://www.ncbi.nlm.nih.gov/pubmed/22005430

shown in numerous studies to induce pathological insulin resistance. Now, to be clear, we are *not* saying, "fats are the cause of insulin resistance." Absolutely not. As will be explained in the next section, no specific macronutrient or subtype of macronutrient is the major cause of insulin resistance. But in extremely high doses, fats and fructose can contribute to it. But again, the reality is that *no macronutrient*—not fats, and not carbs/sugars—is the major culprit of insulin resistance. This section was simply meant to point out the silliness of those trying to demonize sugar (or fructose) on the basis that it damages insulin sensitivity, while simultaneously advocating a way of eating for which there is stronger evidence supporting a role in the development of insulin resistance.

Fructose has been demonized by low-carb gurus extensively in recent years, with some suggesting that not only is it unhealthy, but that it is actually toxic!

There are a couple of very important things to point out about the demonization of fructose:

1) Most of the research used to demonize fructose is research done with rodents, and rodents process fructose in radically different ways than humans do: "Studies that have traced fructose's fantastic voyage through the human body suggest that the liver converts as much as 50 percent of fructose into glucose, around 30 percent of fructose into lactate and less than one percent into fats. In contrast, mice and rats turn more than 50 percent of fructose into fats, so experiments with these animals would exaggerate the significance of fructose's proposed detriments for humans, especially clogged arteries, fatty livers and insulin resistance."[250]
2) The most critical distinction when it comes to fructose—and all the claims of "toxicity" around it—is the *dose*. Countless substances—including those that are *essential* for health and even *survival*—become toxic at certain doses. Virtually all of the studies showing deleterious effects of fructose consumption are from studies where animals are fed an amount of fructose far beyond anything comparable to what the average human consumes.

250 http://blogs.scientificamerican.com/WSS/post.php?blog=61&post=961

As an example of why the dose is so critical to consider in any discussion of whether a specific substance causes insulin resistance, consider this: It is possible to find studies that show that high doses of both *protein* and *fat* cause insulin resistance, just as fructose does. For example:

> "Dietary proteins and amino acids are important modulators of glucose metabolism and insulin sensitivity. Although high intake of dietary proteins has positive effects on energy homeostasis by inducing satiety and possibly increasing energy expenditure, **it has detrimental effects on glucose homeostasis by promoting insulin resistance** and increasing gluconeogenesis."[251]

> "Consumption of energy-dense/high-fat diets is strongly and positively associated with overweight that, in turn, deteriorates insulin sensitivity, particularly when the excess of body fat is located in [the] abdominal region. Nevertheless, the link between fat intake and overweight is not limited to the high energy content of fatty foods; the ability to oxidize dietary fat is impaired in some individuals genetically predisposed to obesity. Insulin sensitivity is also affected by the quality of dietary fat, independently of its effects on body weight. **Epidemiological evidence and intervention studies clearly show that in humans saturated fat significantly worsens insulin resistance**…"[252]

> "**We conclude that high-fat feeding results in insulin resistance**." [253]

> "**Most, although not all, studies suggest that higher levels of total fat in the diet result in greater whole-body insulin resistance**."[254]

Moreover, as pointed out in the introduction of this book, every essential nutrient of life becomes toxic in high doses—sunlight can give you cancer, and water can give you irreversible brain damage or even kill you within hours if you drink too much. Likewise,

---

251 http://www.ncbi.nlm.nih.gov/pubmed/17666010

252 http://www.ncbi.nlm.nih.gov/pubmed/15297079

253 http://classic.ajpendo.physiology.org/content/251/5/E576.short

254 http://www.ncbi.nlm.nih.gov/pubmed/12643169

carbohydrates, protein, and fat can all become harmful at extreme doses. So before we rush to demonize substances, we must take the dose into account.

Consider this quote from David Katz, MD:

> "The levels of fructose intake invoked to produce end-organ damage in provocative articles do not occur under real-world conditions. **Pushed to comparable extremes of dosing, articles about oxygen would reach far grimmer conclusions, concluding the compound is not just toxic, but uniformly lethal over a span of mere days."**[255]

Our purpose here is specifically to address the claims around fructose and insulin resistance, but if you want to explore the specific debates around fructose and its physiological effects, we recommend reading a few articles by nutrition expert Alan Aragon. (Note that Robert Lustig—the world's foremost demonizer of fructose—actually shows up in the comment section of some of those articles for some interesting discussion.)

To bring this back to insulin resistance specifically, for now the important thing to realize is that every macronutrient can cause insulin resistance if the dose is high enough, but *no single macronutrient*—not carbs (nor sugar/fructose), and not fat—nor any macronutrient ratio is the major cause of insulin resistance.

255 http://www.realclearscience.com/blog/2014/10/sugar_is_not_toxic.html

What Happens if You Administer a High-Carbohydrate Diet to Type II Diabetics?

One area where low-carb diets are especially claimed to be important—or even as a necessity—is for those with type II diabetes. Of course, if one is operating on the notion that it is carbohydrates that cause insulin resistance, it would indeed make sense that administering a diet high in carbohydrates to people who are already insulin resistant would be a bad idea.

Yet, as we've already found out, the notion that carbohydrates cause insulin resistance is wrong.

Having said that, we do have studies indicating that some types of low-carb diets can dramatically improve markers of insulin sensitivity. [256] [257] [258]

So, is carbohydrate restriction a necessity for those with insulin resistance/type II diabetes? What really happens when a well-designed high-carbohydrate diet is administered to type II diabetics?

Well, it's certainly not what low-carb gurus expect.

The simple reality is that people have confused causing a temporary rise in blood sugar with chronic hyperglycemia (high blood glucose and insulin resistance), and they are completely different things. Not only that, but well-designed high-carbohydrate diets have the ability to dramatically lower the level of fasting insulin. According to Joel Fuhrman, MD:

> "Probably every nutritional scientist and physician in America knows that insulin levels and insulin resistance parallel body weight. That is basic Physiology 101. … So, it is certainly true—as the advocates of animal-food-rich diets, such as Atkins, Heller, Sears, and other proclaim—carbohydrates drive up insulin levels temporarily. These writers, however, have not presented the data in accurate fashion. **A diet revolving around unrefined carbohydrates (fruits, vegetables, whole grains, and legumes) will not raise blood sugars or insulin levels. Studies**

---

256 http://www.nutritionandmetabolism.com/content/2/1/34

257 http://www.ncbi.nlm.nih.gov/pubmed/16403234

258 http://www.ncbi.nlm.nih.gov/pmc/articles/PMC2633336/

> **have shown that such a diet can reduce fasting insulin levels 30-40 percent in just three weeks.**"[259]

As a matter of fact, there are several studies showing that administering a very high-carbohydrate diet (over 70% carbohydrates, which is significantly *higher* than the roughly 50% carbohydrate diet consumed by most Americans) to people who already have insulin resistance can actually *reverse* insulin resistance!

Neal Barnard, MD's research showed profound reversal of insulin resistance on a 75% carbohydrate vegan diet.[260] Fasting serum glucose dropped by 28% in just 22 weeks on the diet.

Two other studies known as the "Ma Pi" studies [261] [262] took type II diabetics and put them on a 2,200-calorie diet with 70% of calories coming from carbohydrates, which equates to nearly 400g of carbohydrates per day. Interestingly, one of the studies reported on the baseline diet of the participants. Their baseline diet was slightly *lower* in calories (1936 vs. 2174) and considerably *lower in carbohydrate (242 g vs. 392 g)*, which worked out to be 50% carb, 30% fat, and 20% protein.[263] Basically, they did the opposite of what some of the low-carb approaches do—they increased carbohydrate consumption by 20% and decreased fat consumption. Nevertheless, the results of these studies showed improvements that not only rival but surpass the improvements in insulin sensitivity that are seen in many low-carb studies. In the second study, insulin was lowered extremely quickly. And **in the first study, the results were almost unbelievable:**[264]

- **ALL participants were taking insulin prior to starting the diet**
- **ALL no longer required insulin after six months on the diet**

---

259 Fuhrman, J. (2014) The End of Diabetes

260 (http://care.diabetesjournals.org/content/29/8/1777.full)

261 http://medicc.org/mediccreview/articles/mr_119.pdf

262 Medium- and Short-Term Interventions with Ma-Pi 2 Macrobiotic Diet in Type 2 Diabetic Adults of Bauta, Havana.

263 Medium- and Short-Term Interventions with Ma-Pi 2 Macrobiotic Diet in Type 2 Diabetic Adults of Bauta, Havana.

264 http://medicc.org/mediccreview/articles/mr_119.pdf

- **ALL were consuming nearly 400 grams carbohydrate (mostly starch) per day**
- **75% of participants no longer required medications after six months on the diet**

Keep in mind that, in this study, we're talking primarily older women (avg. age 60) who had diabetes for 9 to 31 years, *not* newly diagnosed cases.

Simply put, well-designed high-carbohydrate diets can reverse insulin resistance as well or better than many low-carbohydrate diet interventions.

It is also worth noting that one factor that gets in the way of an accurate analysis of how dietary macronutrient profile impacts insulin sensitivity is whether the diet they are put on is lower in total calories. Any diet—regardless of whether it is very high in carbs or very low in carbs, or very high in fat or very low in fat—will result in profound improvements in insulin sensitivity if it restricts overall caloric intake and causes weight loss. That is, **the fat loss itself will greatly improve insulin sensitivity, regardless of dietary composition.** Lowered calorie intake (and the resultant fat loss) is therefore a major confounding variable that prevents one from drawing conclusions about how dietary composition affects insulin sensitivity.

In fact, in studies where low-carb diets improved insulin sensitivity more than diets higher in carbohydrates, it is frequently the case that the low-carb group simply lost more weight. (Going back to the previous chapter, this effect is driven primarily by higher protein intake and lower food reward/palatability on low-carb diets driving overall calorie intake down more.) This higher level of weight loss will improve insulin sensitivity in and of itself, so in these specific studies, we don't necessarily know whether the improvement was from carbohydrate restriction or simply from calorie restriction.

However, with one of the above Ma Pi studies, they actually *increased* overall calorie intake from the participants' baseline diet. Thus, high-carbohydrate diets can clearly improve insulin sensitivity even in the absence of caloric restriction. The authors of the study concluded, "The higher energy intake observed during this intervention, in comparison to previous values, would indicate that other dietary factors as energy alone should be related to the results. **This Cuban study shows a diet low in fat (only 16–18% of the daily energy),**

low in proteins (12%), and high in whole grain cereals carbohydrates (70–72%) acting alone as powerful medication."[265]

In addition, a study by Dr. Iris Shai et al. found that, **despite eating about the same number of total calories but far *more carbohydrates* than the low-carb group, the Mediterranean diet group lost more weight and had larger improvements in their fasting insulin levels and insulin sensitivity than the low-carb group.**[266] [267]

The question then is whether low-carb interventions improve insulin sensitivity due to being low in carbohydrates or simply due to consuming fewer overall calories and losing body fat. To find the answer to this important question, we need to look at well-controlled studies that test insulin sensitivity on low-carb and higher-carb diets of equal calories. Fortunately, this study has actually been done: Data from a **comprehensive review of calorie-controlled studies that compared the effects on insulin sensitivity of calorie-matched low-carb and high-carb diets found *no benefit whatsoever* from carbohydrate restriction.**[268]

Being generous, we could then conclude that if carbohydrate restriction has some unique metabolic effect separate from the overall calories consumed on a diet, it is such a weak effect that a comprehensive review of calorie-controlled studies can't even detect it.

Thus, based on this research showing that carbohydrate consumption has basically no relationship to insulin resistance, when individual studies that purport to be comparing the effects on insulin resistance of different diets show some advantage for one diet or another, those differences that appear are likely due not to the carbohydrate to fat ratio of that diet, but more to overall food quality and total calories consumed on that diet. Unlike carbohydrate to fat ratios, the evidence is very clear that higher food quality and weight

---

265 http://medicc.org/mediccreview/articles/mr_119.pdf

266 http://www.nejm.org/doi/pdf/10.1056/NEJMoa0708681

267 http://carbsanity.blogspot.com.au/2010/09/shai-and-diabetes.html

268 (http://www.plosone.org/article/info%3Adoi%2F10.1371%2Fjournal.pone.0100652)

loss induced by the consumption of fewer calories are very powerful predictors of the benefit of a given diet.

Not only do studies prove that ingesting carbohydrates does not cause insulin resistance, but there is evidence showing that a well-designed whole foods diet of almost entirely carbohydrates can dramatically *reverse* insulin resistance. These high-carbohydrate diets have been proven to work as well as, or better than, the low-carb diets used in trials with diabetics. Thus, there is no clear evidence that low-carb diets are superior to well-designed higher-carbohydrate diets for improving insulin sensitivity or preventing or reversing type II diabetes. And there is good evidence that well-designed high-carbohydrate diets are at least as effective as many low-carb diets in reversing insulin resistance. However, the most important factors in the diet that relate to insulin resistance are overall food quality and overall calories consumed, and thus the amount of body fat lost—not the macronutrient composition of the diet.

Insulin resistance and type II diabetes are not caused by spiking insulin through eating carbohydrates.

The carbohydrate theory of insulin resistance is simply wrong.

So What Really Causes Insulin Resistance and Type II Diabetes?

First of all, let's get clear on what insulin resistance actually is. Low-carb gurus often portray the fundamental problem as simply a pathologically high excess of insulin (i.e., the problem is that there's too much insulin). And they often conflate this claim of insulin "excess" with the notion that excess insulin is caused by eating too many carbs (i.e., spiking insulin too much). For example, remember those two quotes I shared with you earlier from Mark Hyman, MD and Gary Taubes?

Here is what Mark Hyman says: "Insulin resistance is a condition where you develop a tolerance to insulin and produce excess amounts of insulin. Generally this is because you eat too many sugars or bad carbs."[269] And Taubes' quote: "Anything that increases insulin, induces insulin resistance, and induces the pancreas to compensate by secreting still more insulin, will also lead to an excess accumulation of body fat." [270]

As we've already seen from the previous chapters, this way of portraying what insulin resistance is and what causes it is completely wrong. Insulin resistance/type II diabetes is not a condition where your body is producing "too much insulin," and furthermore, insulin resistance is not caused by "eating too many bad carbs" or eating things that "increase insulin." These statements are not based on any sort of scientific data—they are just plain wrong.

Insulin resistance/type II diabetes is not a state of producing "excess" or "too much" insulin—to the contrary, the body is producing the appropriate amount of insulin to compensate for the real problem. Nor is this—as many people like to conceptualize it—a problem of "too much sugar in the blood." The high blood sugar is not the problem—this too is a *symptom* of the real problem.

The fundamental defect causing insulin resistance is that as body fat mass increases, it becomes harder for the body to restrain all those fat cells from dumping their fatty contents into the blood, and thus insulin is increased as a compensatory response to try to prevent

---

269 Hyman, M. UltraMetabolism.

270 Taubes, G. Good Calories, Bad Calories.

massive increases in blood fatty acids.[271] This increase in body fat leads to the problem of insulin not being able to fully restrain lipolysis and gluconeogenesis, [272] thus leading to the *symptoms* of having high blood sugar levels and the body having to chronically elevate insulin levels.

As Guyenet explains it:

> **"High circulating insulin is probably an adaptive response to insulin resistance in the body, which develops as fat cells enlarge and become less effective at trapping fatty acids and keeping them where they should be (there may also be a contribution from inflammation that may or may not be independent of the changes in fatty acid handling). Elevated insulin is probably the body's way of trying to compensate for this defect and keep fat in fat cells, but it does not fully compensate for the insulin resistance in fat tissue that progressively develops as fat cells enlarge."**[273]

The wording here is critical, because otherwise it's possible to become confused about what the actual problem is in insulin resistance/type II diabetes. This is not a problem where the fundamental pathology is "too much blood sugar" or "too much insulin." These are all *symptoms of the real problem.*

Here is the real chain of causation at work, according to numerous lines of evidence:[274]

---

271 http://carbsanity.blogspot.com/2013/10/the-cause-of-hyperglycemia-in-type-2.html

272 http://diabetes.diabetesjournals.org/content/58/12/2766.full

273 http://wholehealthsource.blogspot.com/2011/09/fat-tissue-insulin-sensitivity-and.html

274 http://wholehealthsource.blogspot.com/2012/12/is-it-time-to-re-write-textbooks-on_13.html

The Chain of Causation in Insulin Resistance

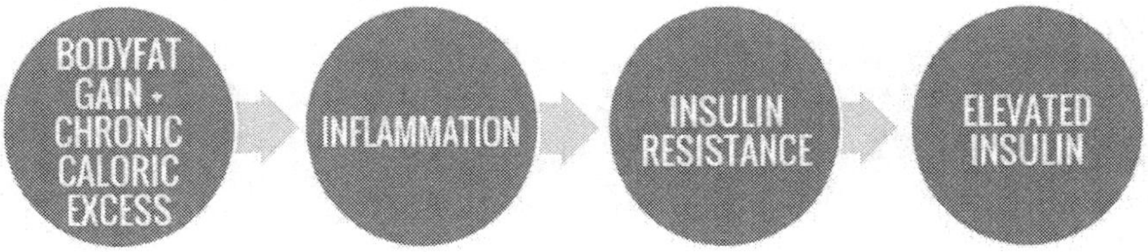

Thus, body fat accumulation causes insulin resistance—not the other way around.

This is why the epidemic of diabetes corresponds extremely well to obesity epidemics but does *not* correspond in any way to cultures consuming higher proportions of their diet from carbohydrate.

Moreover, the simple fact that insulin resistance can be reversed very effectively by losing body fat itself—by following any number of a wide range of diets of widely varying macronutrient profiles—again tells us that the chain of causation goes from body fat gain to insulin resistance, not from insulin resistance to fat gain.[275]

If carbohydrates were the cause of insulin resistance, then the most powerful predictor of improved insulin sensitivity would be carbohydrate restriction (in the absence of fat loss), yet this is not the case—**body fat loss on any type of diet is far more powerful a treatment than simple carbohydrate restriction.**

Now that we understand that insulin resistance is not a problem of "too much sugar" or "too much insulin," let's explore what really causes insulin resistance and type II diabetes.

Guyenet has actually done an in-depth review of the scientific literature on the subject and formulated a comprehensive list of the factors that contribute to insulin resistance:

"These are the factors I'm aware of that can contribute to insulin resistance, listed in approximate order of importance:

---

275 http://wholehealthsource.blogspot.com/2011/09/fat-tissue-insulin-sensitivity-and.html

1) Cellular energy excess
2) Physical inactivity (related to #1)
3) Inflammation (related to #1 and others)
4) Very low carbohydrate intake (less than 10%)
5) Genetics
6) Insulin resistance in the brain
7) Low birth weight/size
8) Inappropriate micronutrient status and insufficient protective phytochemical intake
9) Smoking tobacco
10) High-heat cooking
11) Excessive physical or psychological stress" [276]

Did you notice anything conspicuously absent from that list? Carbohydrates!

If carbohydrates or sugars were *the* primary cause of insulin resistance (or even *a* cause), such a link would be incredibly easy to demonstrate in scientific research. Yet, the studies that have been done on this subject clearly show that this is not the case.

Neither a high-carbohydrate diet nor a high-sugar diet even make it into the top eleven causes of insulin resistance. That's a fairly noteworthy fact considering the number of popular health gurus who are telling people that diabetes is "caused by eating too many sugars and bad carbs" or "insulin resistance is caused by anything that increases insulin."

By far, the single most important cause of insulin resistance is cellular energy excess.

What does that mean? Well, in simple terms, it means *chronic overconsumption of calories.*

This chronic overconsumption of calories is itself highly toxic to the cells. Nutrients in the bloodstream are meant to be kept within a narrow range, and if they get either too low or too high, it can damage the health of the cells. Thus, when there is a chronic excess of nutrients in the blood, it is toxic to the cells.

If you understand physiology fairly well, you might be asking, "But isn't this the reason we have body fat—when there is an excess of nutrients in the blood, the excess will be converted into triglycerides

276 http://wholehealthsource.blogspot.com/2012/01/what-causes-insulin-resistance-part-vii.html

and stored as body fat, thus allowing nutrients in the blood to be kept in their optimal ranges?"

And this is indeed true! **The problem is that when there is a *chronic* overconsumption of calories and a significant increase in body fatness (i.e., the person becomes overweight or obese), the body becomes *less efficient* at mopping up the excess nutrients by shuttling them into body fat stores, and the result is chronically elevated levels of nutrients floating around in the blood.**

If the cells were in their normal state of letting nutrients into the cell with ease, they would quickly be flooded with nutrients and would become toxic. So the cells actually respond to this chronic overabundance of nutrients in the blood by going into an intelligent and adaptive insulin resistance—they are trying to *protect* themselves from the toxicity of the overabundance of nutrients (fats and glucose) in the blood by becoming insulin resistant and taking in less of those nutrients. (Note: This is true more so with glucose because of down-regulating the GLUT4 glucose transporters, but the problem is the cells *can't* really prevent the fatty acids from entering as these are soluble in cell membranes and can pass through them, and thus do build up in the cells. This is actually what led Neal Barnard, MD, to theorize that buildup of intramyocellular lipid is the fundamental cause of insulin resistance, which is likely why he believed—incorrectly—that the cause is dietary fat consumption, and the *only* solution is to eat a low-fat vegetarian diet.)

Insulin resistance is an intelligent and adaptive response (i.e., not a pathological response) to a chronic overconsumption of calories, which is the real pathology. Insulin levels tend to parallel bodyweight, but it's not because higher levels of insulin make you fatter (as many low-carb gurus believe)—it's because *both* body fat gain and insulin resistance are driven by the same thing, which is chronic overconsumption of calories. Moreover, as a person gets fatter, their fat cells do their job of mopping up nutrient excess less efficiently, and insulin levels rise as a side effect of being overweight, not the other way around. In addition, when body fat increases to a certain level, insulin is not able to do its job of keeping fat in the cells (restraining lipolysis), and as a result, blood fats build up and cause further problems. In simple terms, low-carb gurus have become confused about the chain of causation in insulin resistance in their attempts to blame things on carbohydrates and insulin themselves. The fundamental problem isn't carbohydrates—it's chronic calorie overconsumption and body fat gain.

Beyond chronic calorie overconsumption and body fat gain—which are the most important causes of insulin resistance—there are numerous other factors linked to insulin resistance:

Lack of exercise or "inactivity": Exercise (or "activity") is a factor that sensitizes the cells to insulin. Similarly, lack of exercise can, over time, promote insulin resistance.

Sitting: Separate from, and even more important than, lack of exercise, the act of prolonged sitting itself can induce profound insulin resistance in shockingly short periods of time. This is a major cause of insulin resistance in those who work desk jobs sitting in front of a computer for eight or ten hours each day. Studies have shown that just a single day of inactivity can cause a shocking amount of insulin resistance.[277]

Inflammation: Inflammation from various sources like inflammatory and allergenic foods can induce insulin resistance very powerfully. And anti-inflammatories such as aspirin-related compounds have proven to have remarkable effects on reducing insulin resistance.[278]

Genetics and low birth weight: Both of these can predispose one to higher risk for insulin resistance and type II diabetes, such that when environmental factors like chronic overconsumption of calories and sedentariness are present, they will be more likely to become insulin resistant and/or diabetic.[279]

High-heat cooking: This has been shown to create cooking byproducts that worsen insulin sensitivity.[280]

---

277 http://blogs.plos.org/obesitypanacea/2012/04/04/sitting-for-just-a-couple-hours-has-measurable-and-negative-health-impact/

278 http://wholehealthsource.blogspot.com/2012/01/what-causes-insulin-resistance-part-vii.html

279 http://wholehealthsource.blogspot.com/2012/01/what-causes-insulin-resistance-part-vii.html

280 http://wholehealthsource.blogspot.com/2012/01/what-causes-insulin-resistance-part-vii.html

Smoking: This can also cause insulin resistance.[281]

Intense or prolonged elevated levels of stress hormones: This impairs the body's ability to suppress glucose production when it is already plentiful.[282]

Extremely *low*-carbohydrate diets: In direct contradiction to the common belief that high carbohydrate intakes cause insulin resistance and low carbohydrate intakes prevent it, very low-carbohydrate diets can induce insulin resistance.[283] But this is largely an adaptive (i.e., not a pathological) insulin resistance. Why does the body become insulin resistant on extremely low-carbohydrate diets? Well, glucose (i.e., sugar) is the preferred, and generally the only, fuel source of the brain. The brain can use ketones to some degree in a state of starvation or an extreme low-carbohydrate diet, but in general, for 99.999999% of people who are in a normal state of physiology, their brains are running on sugar. When one goes on a diet where sugar/carbohydrates are present only in very small amounts, the body intelligently goes into a state of whole-body insulin resistance to prevent muscles and organs from using up the sugar that is present so that as much sugar as possible can go to feed the body's most important organ—the brain.

Micronutrient deficiency: Micronutrients, such as magnesium for example, are a massive factor in insulin resistance.[284] One study has illustrated just how important optimal magnesium status is: they put people on a low-magnesium diet (and by the way, the typical Western diet is magnesium deficient) and showed that the diet increased insulin resistance by a whopping 25% in just 3 weeks.[285] This means that just 3 weeks of taking in very little of this one micronutrient significantly damaged the body's ability to efficiently regulate nutrients from the blood. Numerous other vitamins, minerals, and phytonutrients exert an impact on insulin sensitivity

281 http://wholehealthsource.blogspot.com/2012/01/what-causes-insulin-resistance-part-vii.html

282 http://press.endocrine.org/doi/abs/10.1210/jcem-54-1-131

283 http://wholehealthsource.blogspot.com/2012/01/what-causes-insulin-resistance-part-vii.html

284 http://care.diabetesjournals.org/content/28/5/1175.full

285 http://hyper.ahajournals.org/content/21/6_Pt_2/1024.full.pdf

as well. This is a major reason why consuming a diet rich in processed foods—which are typically deficient in micronutrients—can predispose one to insulin resistance.

Some other possible causes of insulin resistance:

- Binge drinking[286]
- Lack of sleep[287]
- Exercise-induced muscle damage[288]
- Hormonal imbalance such as PCOS or estrogen dominance
- Food additives like BPA and carrageenan[289] [290]
- Endotoxin leaking into the bloodstream due to gut permeability[291] [292]
- Gut dysbiosis[293]
- Glycine deficiency[294]
- Trans-fat consumption[295]
- Hypothyroidism[296]

Now let's imagine a scenario:

√ Let's put someone on a diet that is magnesium-deficient—not just for three weeks like the above study, but for two decades.

√ Let's add in plenty of high-heat cooking and fried foods high in trans-fats.

---

286 http://www.medicalnewstoday.com/articles/255716.php

287 http://www.precisionnutrition.com/sleep-and-insulin-resistance

288 http://www.ncbi.nlm.nih.gov/pubmed/1629073

289 http://www.ncbi.nlm.nih.gov/pmc/articles/PMC1332699/

290 http://www.ncbi.nlm.nih.gov/pubmed/22011715

291 http://diabetes.diabetesjournals.org/content/56/7/1761.full

292 http://www.ncbi.nlm.nih.gov/pubmed/11050051

293 http://www.ncbi.nlm.nih.gov/pubmed/20140211

294 https://www.bcm.edu/news/geriatrics/glutathione-deficiency-fat-insulin-aging

295 http://www.ncbi.nlm.nih.gov/pubmed/17636085

296 http://www.ncbi.nlm.nih.gov/pmc/articles/PMC3356957/

- √ Let's add in a desk job that requires this person to sit for eight hours each day, and then when they come home from work, they sit in front of the TV for another couple of hours.
- √ Let's throw in a really high omega-6 fat intake from vegetable oils to disrupt the omega-6 to omega-3 ratio and promote inflammation.
- √ Let's add a stressful job or personal life into the mix.
- √ Maybe throw in some occasional binge drinking and consuming foods laced with BPA.
- √ Then, let's add chronically disrupted sleep/circadian rhythm.
- √ Finally, let's add in lots of highly rewarding processed foods that drive chronic overconsumption of calories and fat gain.

All of these factors have by themselves proven to induce insulin resistance. Combine several of them together—as is common for modern Westerners—and you now have the perfect storm of over a dozen different factors for creating insulin resistance/type II diabetes. And all of a sudden, it becomes obvious why there is a diabetes epidemic in the United States—and it has little to do with sugars or "bad carbs."

Carbohydrates—even refined carbohydrates and sugar—are not the cause of insulin resistance.

If you have insulin resistance/type II diabetes or are looking to prevent it, our suggestion is to address the above listed fifteen or so factors implicated in insulin resistance as well as your overall body fat percentage, rather than concern yourself with carbohydrates.

All of the factors mentioned above are infinitely more important than the carbohydrate to fat ratio of your diet.

Get processed foods out of your diet; move your body and do ample exercise; if you work a desk job, then get a standing desk or treadmill desk; don't smoke or drink excessively; take measures for destressing, like yoga or meditation; normalize your circadian rhythm; heal your gut function and bacterial profile; address any hormonal imbalances you have; correct your thyroid and metabolic function; and eat a diet high in vitamin-rich and mineral-rich animal and plant foods to make sure you have an abundance of micronutrients and phytonutrients. In general, eat a nutrient-dense whole-food diet. Most importantly, lose body fat, for that is the most powerful way to re-establish healthy insulin sensitivity. These strategies are likely to enhance your health and insulin sensitivity far more powerfully than simply restricting the amount of carbohydrates in your diet.

SUMMARY

If carbohydrates or sugar were a major cause of insulin resistance, this effect would be incredibly easy to demonstrate in a scientific study. Just as numerous studies have easily demonstrated that increased body fat mass causes insulin resistance, that magnesium deficiency causes insulin resistance, that sleep deprivation causes insulin resistance, and that sitting for prolonged periods causes insulin resistance, so too, if the low-carb gurus are right about carbohydrates causing insulin resistance, this should be an incredibly easy thing to demonstrate in a scientific study. Yet, dozens of studies show no such link. At best, we are talking about extremely weak evidence of any link.

If carbohydrates were making people insulin resistant, it would also be very easy to prove that reversing insulin resistance is only possible on low-carb diets, and that low-carb diets are far and away superior to any sort of high-carbohydrate diet. Yet the studies do *not* show this.

In general, the research indicates that low-carb and high-carb diets—when factors such as total calorie intake, fat loss, and overall food quality of the diet are accounted for—are about equally as effective in reversing type II diabetes/insulin resistance. Insulin resistance can be reversed very effectively from following any number of diets of high food quality that vary wildly in terms of carbohydrate to fat ratio.

Moreover, if carbohydrates (and the simple act of eating foods that cause insulin secretion) were the cause of insulin resistance, then administering any sort of high-carbohydrate diet to type II diabetics would make their insulin resistance worse, not better. Yet, we have numerous studies showing this isn't true, and that well-designed high-carbohydrate diets can not only control insulin resistance, but actually *reverse* it!

To summarize everything we've gone over here:

- Dietary carbohydrate does not cause insulin resistance or diabetes.
- Carbohydrate restriction and low-carb diets are absolutely not necessary to reverse insulin resistance. As much research has

proven, very high-carb diets like the Ma Pi diets can reverse insulin resistance as well or better than low-carb diets.

- The main effect of a particular diet reversing insulin resistance is driven by overall fat loss (due to decreased calorie consumption)—not by the inherent metabolic effects of a diet's macronutrient content.
- Diabetes epidemics can occur without any parallel increase in carbohydrate consumption.
- Studies testing if carbohydrate consumption in healthy people causes insulin resistance show that it does not lead to insulin resistance/diabetes.
- Studies testing if high-glycemic sugars cause insulin resistance in healthy people show that they have shown extremely weak evidence that sugar is a major cause of insulin resistance.
- Numerous studies have shown improved insulin sensitivity and reduced fasting insulin as a result of eating very-high-carbohydrate diets. Numerous of these studies have proven that high-carbohydrate diets can be just as effective a treatment for type II diabetics as any low-carb diet.
- We can find numerous populations around the world eating a diet of far *more* carbohydrate than the amount of carbohydrate consumed in populations that have diabetes epidemics, and yet, these populations have negligible to no insulin resistance/type II diabetes.
- The only sugar that is in any way linked with insulin resistance is fructose. Yet, to actually get insulin resistance from fructose consumption, it requires intake of extreme amounts of fructose well beyond what almost any normal individual would ever consume. While sugar-sweetened beverages are best avoided due to their role in promoting fat gain and the associated insulin resistance, fruit consumption is linked with *improved*, not worsened, insulin sensitivity.
- The epidemic of insulin resistance/type II diabetes is caused by a combination of factors—primarily chronic overconsumption of calories, sitting and inactivity, inflammation, genetic predisposition, high-heat cooking, smoking, stress, lack of sleep, gut bacteria imbalance, hypothyroidism, and

> micronutrient and phytonutrient deficiencies. It is *not* caused by carbohydrates.

None of this is to say that low-carb diets *don't* work or are "bad." There is actually much research indicating that they are one effective potential approach, and that they work about as well as any other whole-food diets of equal calories. But it is to say that carbohydrates are not the cause of insulin resistance, and low-carb diets are not necessary to reverse insulin resistance.

Simply put, everywhere we might look to find evidence validating the idea that carbohydrates—even high-glycemic carbohydrates—lead to insulin resistance and type II diabetes, the evidence is extremely weak.

Carbohydrate consumption is not the cause of insulin resistance/type II diabetes.

Chapter 5: Fats - The Fuel of Superhuman Athletes or Athletes Who Can Barely Keep Up?

Outside of the vast internet- and book-based world of nutrition advice, there exists the practical world of sport and athletics. While many nutrition gurus portray athletes as "bad examples" because they "eat whatever they want," the reality is that sport is Darwinian. If eating a certain way gave definitive performance enhancement, that way would be well known and well favored. Let us remember that during the Soviet era, huge government-funded organizations in the Eastern bloc countries employed high-level PhD and MD research scientists to figure out anything that would give their athletes an edge. From this research came the explosion of Performance Enhancing Drugs (PEDs), notably anabolic steroids, growth hormone, cortisol and insulin injections, EPO, blood doping, and lesser-known drugs. Color therapy, diet manipulation, oxygen water, hyperbaric chambers, hypnosis, yoga techniques, ice baths, compression stockings, creative visualization, and many other techniques were all examined in detail by the Soviet bloc's athletic development programs. While many of these proved to be highly effective and are now part of the everyday practice of athletic performance, radical manipulation of carbohydrate to fat ratio of the diet has proven to be of minimal value.

Instead, a growing body of research has examined over time the diet needs of sports as diverse as marathon running and pro football and come up repeatedly with the same conclusions: athletes perform best when they eat a well-balanced diet with sufficient protein, fat, and carbohydrates so that they can fuel their training and recovery. For virtually every sport or training activity, carbohydrates play a large and critical role as a primary fuel for exercise and recovery.

We must remember that at the peak of competitive athletics, athletes will do just about *anything* to get an extra edge over their competition—including illegal drugs, blood doping, substances that will lead to them being banned from competition for life, and playing with all sorts of chemicals that have totally unknown long-term health effects. Untold amounts of money and time are spent taking such substances and then hiding their use from the governing authorities of their sport. The simple fact is that, when it comes down to it, athletes will do just about *anything* to win—including things that may end up being extremely damaging to their health. If a high-level coach told his athletes that drinking gasoline before each race would improve their performance, most elite athletes would do it. That's how extreme the desire to win is among elite athletes. Thus, if something as *un-extreme* as eating a low-carb, high-fat diet reliably provided any sort of even meager performance advantage, this way of eating would be standard practice.

This is precisely the reason that low-carb diets are virtually never found among elite competitors, no matter the sport—because it doesn't enhance performance.

Yet, in recent years, there has been an unhealthful and scientifically ridiculous trend towards advising hard exercisers to try to become "fat-adapted" to improve their performance and reduce body fat. (For example, Peter Attia has a 77-minute lecture on YouTube speaking about it as an "advantaged metabolic state."[297]) Becoming "fat-adapted" means that you train your body to burn fat for fuel instead of its preferred source of fuel, carbohydrates. This is done essentially by avoiding carbohydrates, since as long as you eat ample carbohydrates, the body will preferentially use carbohydrates for fuel. But it also involves restricting protein as well, since a high protein intake will also prevent you from getting into ketosis and becoming fully fat-adapted. The "how to" of becoming fat-adapted sounds simple enough but appears in practice to be quite difficult and

297 https://www.youtube.com/watch?v=NqwvcrA7oe8

impractical. Several of these low-carb endurance athlete advocates explain in great and painful detail on their websites how to stay in ketosis or near ketosis, how to get through the feelings of weakness, headaches, and constipation, and how easily their fat-burning state gets thrown off if they eat something like an apple or a couple of carrots.

Nonetheless, by strictly limiting both carbohydrates and protein, and eating a diet typically of at least 65% fat, you can indeed enter the mythical state of being "fat-adapted." As a result of becoming fat-adapted, the low-carb gurus claim that your body fat starts to get used for energy instead of just sitting on your body and making you look bad, and you have miraculous amounts of unlimited energy. You never tire. You never crash. You can perform forever!

Or so the claims go…

Fortunately, some of the greatest endurance athletes in the world such as the Kenyan distance runners and Tarahumara Indian ultradistance runners have never read about the "amazing benefits" of being in ketosis or becoming "fat-adapted."

The Kenyans own practically every distance record and major race championship in the past 20 years. So as a good start for examining which dietary pattern is likely ideal for elite endurance performance, let's look at what the Kenyans eat. Lucky for us, their diet has been analyzed extensively by scientists:

Mukeshi and Thairu found that **Kenyan runners consumed an average of 441 grams of carbohydrate daily (with approximately 75% of their total caloric intake coming from carbohydrates).**[298]

Christensen et al studied Kenyan runners from an area of Kenya known as Kilenjin, which produced an incredible 40% of winners of all major international middle- and long-distance running competitions between 1987 and 1997. **These runners consumed an average of 476 grams of carbohydrates daily (71% of total calories).** [299]

Another study detailed their daily diet as consisting of bread, boiled rice, boiled potatoes, porridge, cabbage, kidney beans, and a thick maize meal paste known as ugali, with meat eaten just four times per

298 Mukeshi M, Thairu K. Nutrition and body build: a Kenyan review. World Review of Nutrition and Dietetics, 1993; 72: 218-226.

299 Christensen DL, et al. Food and macronutrient intake of male adolescent Kalenjin runners in Kenya. British Journal of Nutrition, 2002; 88 (6): 711-717.

week, and large amounts of tea with milk and sugar consumed throughout the day. This study found that **total daily carbohydrate intake was 607 grams**, and daily protein and fat intakes were 75 and 45 grams, respectively.[300]

The Tarahumara (their actual name means the running people) routinely run 100- to 300-mile races. **Their diet has been meticulously documented and is approximately 75% carbohydrate,** based mostly on corn, potatoes, squash, and beans.[301] Interestingly, one of the few Westerners to ever beat or keep up with the Tarahumara in a major ultradistance race is the famous ultrarunner, Scott Jurek, who is well known for his tremendous running career and his vegan diet, which, needless to say, is an ultra-high-carbohydrate diet.

Running or endurance exercising on a low-carb, high-fat diet is possible. A variety of studies have shown that in the short term, athletes can adapt and perform and apparently burn more fat and less glycogen for their exercise fuel. However, the effect is inconsistent and unpredictable. In other words, some athletes can do this, but most cannot. And the effect in those who can use fat effectively does not reliably make them faster, stronger, or able to last longer.

What about athletes who rely on feats of strength and power, like so many sports do? Can these athletes become fat-adapted? The answer in plain English is no. They *can* become fat-adapted to the extent that they are burning more fat overall—during rest and times of lower intensity physical activity—but there is simply no way around the basic physiological fact that high-intensity sprint efforts (like the type of efforts most sports rely on to one degree or another) cannot be fueled by fat. The muscles *require* glucose (carbohydrate) for higher-intensity bursts. Athletes or exercisers who require quick movement and contracture of fast twitch (explosive) muscle fibers simply *need* carbohydrates to perform well. Football, hockey, soccer, tennis, spinning class, track, swimming, cycling, boxing and mixed martial arts, and even CrossFit—all of these demand glycogen and carbohydrates for top performance. It's not a case of this being optional where one

---

300 Onywera VO, et al. Food and Macronutrient Intake of EliteKenyan Distance Runners. International Journal of Sport Nutrition and Exercise Metabolism, 2004; 14: 709-719.

301 http://ajcn.nutrition.org/content/32/4/905.full.pdf

can choose whether they want to eat carbs or not eat carbs and they will perform equally well either way—it's a case of "eat ample carbs or you will not be an elite competitor in your sport."

Can you make it through a moderate spinning class without carbs? Sure, but most athletes are not trying to make it through their training or event. They want to improve, compete, and feel better in their activity, not just "get through" because of misguided adherence to an intellectually appealing but physiologically unfruitful diet.

The theory of low-carb eating for athletes never matches the reality. CrossFit advocates a low-carb Paleo diet, which permits consumption of primarily protein and fat while limiting carbohydrate. As detailed in the section of this book on ancestral diets, this concept of the "Paleo" diet is not scientific—it is based on the myth that our prehistoric ancestors were all "fat-burning machines" who ate low-carb diets. The idea is romantic and appealing, yet in discussions with CrossFit competitors and top coaches, the quiet truth is that the typical low-carb Paleo diet is not enough to fuel high-level performance. There is nothing wrong with hard-working athletes and their coaches admitting that they eat peanut butter sandwiches before training or competition, or rice or potatoes or whatever. What is wrong is for commercial interests and low-carb gurus to not admit these facts and to advocate ridiculous diets to the general exercising public that will leave them tired and unhappy.

From time to time, an elite athlete will be in the public eye because they are on the Paleo diet or other carbohydrate-restricted diet. We see interviews on the low-carb websites highlighting their "conversion." Recently, a world champion female rower was on several sites describing her dietary changes and exactly what she was eating. She had gotten rid of grains and starches and said she felt great and was "relearning" how to train on such a diet. Why does a world champion need to relearn how to train in order to follow a diet? Unfortunately, she did not qualify in the following year for her national team and obviously did not improve upon her world championship placing the year before. Her performance decrement, however, was never mentioned in any of the low-carb websites that had so enthusiastically endorsed her at the start. In fact, she was never mentioned again anywhere on a diet website. Occasionally, we also hear from low-carb gurus of one or another athlete who they claim is eating a low-carb diet. Yet, when one looks more deeply into the diets of such athletes, it is often discovered that they aren't nearly as "low-carb" as is claimed.

The point of this is that a few athletes mentioned briefly in the news is not the same as long-term scientific studies examining thousands of athletes over the years. The scientific evidence is clear. More important, the experience of athletes and coaches is clear. If low-carb eating worked, all sports would be pushing it on their athletes. In fact, the NFL and NHL training tables of old used to do exactly that. Steak, eggs, and salad were the staples of the NFL training table. Sport science eventually proved that athletes would perform better with a more carbohydrate-based diet, and the NFL and NHL changed.

Low-carb exercising is not new, and the history is not pretty. In the sixties, with the advent of commercially competitive bodybuilding, high-protein, low-carb diets were advocated to "get cut" (lower body fat to improve muscle definition). A huge industry centered on protein powders and other "necessary" items to burn fat and build muscle was founded and promoted by the muscle magazines. Many bodybuilders were eating 300 to 500 grams of protein per day! These hugely expensive diets resulted in low energy, insomnia, fatigue, and kidney problems. Over time, bodybuilders found that low-carb diets were unsustainable and did not provide enough energy for the highly intense workouts needed to build and sustain muscle mass. According to Dan Gwartney, MD, "Low-carbohydrate diets were seized with glee and zeal initially, particularly among the drug-free crowd as body fat and subcutaneous water are shed with unparalleled results. However, over the years, the low-carbohydrate diets appeared to take their toll on bodybuilders and the sport. From contest to contest, bodybuilders who followed a low-carbohydrate diet progressively lost size, fullness, and presentation; injuries, onstage cramping, and other maladies became prevalent."[302] Today's bodybuilders, whether at the hobby or pro level, include ample carbohydrates in their diet. Many elite competitors eat close to 1,000 grams of carbohydrates daily. There are no examples—that we are aware of—of elite bodybuilders who chronically restrict carbohydrates or who are operating in ketosis all the time. It is common knowledge among elite bodybuilders and their coaches that muscles do not grow as well on low-carb diets. The only

302 http://www.musculardevelopment.com/articles/nutrition/2635-old-school-bodybuilding-carbs-make-a-comeback.html#.VJxIFbjBA

time that low-carb diets are commonly used by bodybuilders is during "cutting" phases where growing muscle isn't a concern like it is for most of year. But even here, many of the most elite bodybuilders are no longer even doing low-carb diets—many still consume well over 400g of carbohydrates per day even up to the day of their show.[303] Elite bodybuilding coaches like Hany Rambod and George Farah work with the best bodybuilders in the world and use high-carbohydrate diets. Bodybuilding is not necessarily the most healthful sport or the most athletic, but when it comes to building muscle mass and lowering body fat, no group on Earth has more expertise. It's not a mistake—or due to their ignorance—that they eat large amounts of carbohydrates.

Carbohydrates are necessary to form glycogen, which is stored in the muscles and liver and is used to fuel high-intensity muscular contractions during exercise. Athletes know this intuitively because if they do not eat adequate carbohydrates, their training and performance suffer. The athlete's intuition is supported by extensive scientific evidence dating back to the research of the Cold War. Overall, the research shows that while it is possible for some endurance athletes to train and thrive on a low-carb diet, most will not. Strength athletes and combination athletes who compete in sports with strength, speed, power, and endurance demands clearly require carbohydrates to obtain high performance levels. Low-carb eating while adhering to an exercise regimen of high-intensity exercises or most competitive athletics is destined to lead to hunger, cravings, low energy, and decreased performance. This is why the great majority of elite and high-level athletes, in virtually all sports, include substantial amounts of carbohydrates in their diet.

Yet, despite all of this history and the simple fact that athletes of virtually all sports have already figured out that they need ample dietary carbs to perform at their best, there are still some researchers, physicians, and various diet guru figures in the low-carb movement who claim that low-carb ketogenic diets are not only healthier, are not only our bodies' "preferred" or "ancestral" physiological state, but also that ketones and fat are superior fuel sources that enhance physical performance.

---

303 http://www.musculardevelopment.com/articles/nutrition/2635-old-school-bodybuilding-carbs-make-a-comeback.html#.VJxIFbjBA

Most often, these recommendations are made for extreme endurance athletes such as long-distance runners and triathletes. However, those recommending these diets frequently extend their advice to all types of athletes and exercisers.

Of course, one can always cherry-pick the data (or shape the data) to give the impression that low-carb diets do improve performance. For example, many low-carb advocates bring up the 1983 study by Phinney et al.[304] as evidence of the efficacy of low-carb eating on athletic performance. And on the surface, this study appears to support the efficacy of low-carb ketogenic diets for endurance since the ketogenic group went an average of four minutes longer in their time-to-exhaustion (TTE) cycling test.

Yet, upon closer inspection, there are some rather important details of this study that the TTE averages don't communicate very well. So let's talk about the details of this study.

First of all, this study involved only five subjects, which is an extremely small number of participants, far too small in fact to be used as a definitive study. (That's an important detail that we'll come back to in a moment.) The way the study was designed was that subjects were first put on a conventional diet and then were put on a ketogenic diet for four weeks thereafter. By the end of the fourth week, the participants were verified (via respiratory quotient, or RQ) to be fat-adapted. Their RQ dropped to 0.72, which is about as fat-adapted as it is possible to be (0.7 would be a pure fat burner, and 1.0 would be a pure carb burner). That's important since many low-carb gurus claim that complete fat-adaptation is necessary to see the so-called "benefits" of ketogenic diets on performance. These subjects were indeed fully fat-adapted.

Now, let's get to the results:

1) Pre-keto (i.e., carbohydrate-based diet) performance at the beginning of the study was *not* significantly different from participants' performance after the ketogenic diet. That's the first critical point here. The overall effect—if one is to say there was any effect—is very small.

---

304 Phinney SD, Bistrian BR, Evans WJ, Gervino E, Blackburn GL. The human metabolic response to chronic ketosis without caloric restriction: preservation of submaximal exercise capability with reduced carbohydrate oxidation. Metabolism. 1983 Aug;32(8):769-76.

2) Mean TTE in the non-keto condition was 147 minutes. TTE in the keto group, after fat-adaptation, was 151 minutes. So it appears, based on this, that the ketogenic diet had a benefit to performance.
3) When we look at the individual TTE of the five participants, we see that two of the five participants experienced massive *declines* in performance (TTE decreased by a whopping 48 minutes and 51 minutes), while one other participant had a 3-minute increase, another one had a 31-minute increase, and one of the five participants had an enormous 84 minute increase in TTE.

The bottom line of this study is that one person had minimal change, half of the remaining four-person group significantly increased their performance (with one of those increasing it enormously and skewing the data), and then the other half of the group dramatically *worsened* their performance.

So what did this study actually tell us?

Well, basically nothing, because the sample size was far too small and the results far too scattered to have any meaning at all. But if you were to draw some kind of conclusion from it (if, say, these same results were found in studies with a lot more participants), you could say that ketogenic diets are likely to either dramatically improve your performance or dramatically worsen it, and you have a roughly equal chance of one of those two things occurring.

What this study most definitely did *not* say is that ketogenic diets are a reliable way to improve performance. Without the one person who had a freakish increase in TTE, the results would have clearly shown negative performance effects.

Moreover, 21 years after the aforementioned study, Phinney actually reflected on the results of his 1983 study and noted:

> "The bicyclist subjects of this study noted a modest decline in their energy level while on training rides during the first week of the Inuit diet, after which subjective **performance was reasonably restored except for their sprint capability, which**

> **remained constrained during the period of carbohydrate restriction."**[305]

This is particularly notable since most sports—virtually all those that are not endurance races—rely on sprint capability, and even Phinney himself acknowledges that sprint capability was significantly impaired.

(Nutrition expert Alan Aragon dissects this study—and many other low-carb arguments—in a debate with low-carb advocate Jeff Volek)

Now, you might be wondering about the performance effects of slightly less extreme carbohydrate restriction. Perhaps that has benefits?

Studies from Jern W. Helge of the University of Copenhagen give us a good answer to that question. He conducted experiments to determine the effects of low-carb, high-fat diets versus high-carb, low-fat diets on endurance performance. **At seven weeks into the study, time to exhaustion was tested, and the high-carb group improved their time by 191 percent compared to only 68 percent in the low-carb group.**[306] In looking at the data, they concluded:

> **"Adaptation to a fat-rich diet, in combination with training, from 1-4 weeks, does not reduce endurance performance compared with a diet rich in carbohydrates, but when dietary treatment and training are continued for 7 weeks, endurance performance is markedly better when a carbohydrate-rich diet is consumed."**[307]

But rather than looking at just one or another study (particularly studies like Phinney's that only had five participants), it is wise to look at the research as a whole to see what the general trend is.

Fortunately for us, Trent Stellingwerff, a physiology researcher at the Canadian Sport Institute, compiled a summary of the 21 English language, peer-reviewed studies that examined the effect of

---

305 Phinney SD. Ketogenic diets and physical performance. Nutr Metab (Lond). 2004 Aug 17;1(1):2.Phinney SD. Ketogenic diets and physical performance. Nutr Metab (Lond). 2004 Aug 17;1(1):2.

306 http://www.ncbi.nlm.nih.gov/pubmed/11103848

307

http://journals.cambridge.org/download.php?file=%2FPNS%2FPNS57_01%2FS0029665198000159a.pdf&code=7a4addf15a6536119ea5704c1f57a0b3

carbohydrate restriction and fat adaptation on athletic performance. He compiled the studies into a table under three columns: those studies that showed a performance decrease, those that showed no effect, and those that showed improved performance. Here is the table the Stellingwerff created:

Published Data –Short to Moderate Term Fat Adaptation or Ketogenic Dietary Impact on Exercise Performance (each individual perf. test per study shown)

Performance Decrease (12)	**No Effect** (7)	**Improved Performance** (2)
Bergstrom, J., et al., Acta Physiologica Scandinavica, 1967. 71(2): p. 140-50.	Phinney, S.D., et al., Metabolism, 1983. 32(8): p. 769-76.	Lambert, E.V., et al., International journal of sport nutrition and exercise metabolism, 2001. 11(2): p. 209-25.
CHRISTENSEN, E. H.,et al., *Scand. Arch. Physiol.* 81:160–171, 1939.	Havemann, L., et al., 100km performance. J Appl Physiol (1985). 2006. 100(1): p. 194-202.	Lambert, E.V., et al., Inc. Perf. Prolonged Test. Eur J Appl Physiol Occup Physiol, 1994. 69(4): p. 287-93.
GALBO, H. et al. *Acta Physiol. Scand.* 107:19–32, 1979.	Burke LM, et al. *J Appl Physiol* 89: 2413–2421, 2000.	
Pitsiladis, Y.P. Et al. The Journal of physiology, 1999. 517 (Pt 3): p. 919-30.	Burke LM, et al., *Med Sci Sports Exerc* 34: 83–91, 2002.	
Starling, R.D., et al., Journal of Applied Physiology, 1997. 82(4): p. 1185-9.	Carey AL,et al. , *J Appl Physiol* 91: 115–122, 2001.	
Maughan, R.J. and D.C. Poole, Eur J Appl Physiol Occup Physiol, 1981. 46(3): p. 211-9.	Lambert, E.V., et al., No Change High Intensity Test. Eur J Appl Physiol Occup Physiol, 1994. 69(4): p. 287-93.	
Greenhaff, P.L., et al. European journal of applied physiology and occupational physiology, 1987. 56(3): p. 331-7.	Goedecke, J.H., et al., Metabolism, 1999. 48(12): p. 1509-17.	
Greenhaff, P.L., et al., European journal of applied physiology and occupational physiology, 1987. 56(4): p. 444-50.		
Greenhaff, P.L., et al. European journal of applied physiology and occupational physiology, 1988. 57(5): p. 583-90.		
Havemann, L., et al., 1k sprint performance. J Appl Physiol (1985). 2006. 100(1): p. 194-202.		
Havemann, L., et al., 4k sprint performance. J Appl Physiol (1985). 2006. 100(1): p. 194-202.		
O'KEEFFE, et al. *Nutr. Res.* 9:819–830, 1989.		

The data is very straightforward: Of the 21 studies, 7 showed minimal or no effects in either direction, 12 studies showed decreased performance, and only 2 showed improvement. [308]

This pretty much speaks for itself. **The data most definitely does *not* indicate that low-carb diets are a good way to improve performance. If anything, the scientific data shows that low-carb diets are a reliable way to *worsen* athletic performance.**

At best, one can make the case that such diets can lead to improved performance in ultra-endurance races while they unquestionably worsen performance in high-intensity efforts that most sports depend on. At worst, they lower performance in every type of activity.

A review of the literature on the effects of high-fat, low-carb diets titled "High-carbohydrate versus high-fat diets in endurance sports" concluded:

---

308 https://twitter.com/TStellingwerff/status/533690289987145729/photo/1

> **"Therefore there is currently very little or no evidence to support the use of high-fat diets and long-term health effects of such diets in athletes are unknown."**[309]

Another review from 2007 titled "Low-carbohydrate diets and performance" had this to say:

"Athletes are continually searching for means to optimize their performance. Within the past 20 years, athletes and scientists have reported or observed that consuming a carbohydrate-restricted diet may improve performance. The original theories explaining the purported benefits centered on the fact that fat oxidation increases, thereby "sparing" muscle glycogen. More recent concepts that explain the plausibility of the ergogenicity of low-carbohydrate, or high-fat, diets on exercise performance pertain to an effect similar to altitude training. **We and others have observed that although fat oxidation may be increased, the ability to maintain high-intensity exercise (above the lactate threshold) seems to be compromised or at least indifferent when compared with consumption of more carbohydrate.**"[310]

According to McArdle et al. in the exercise physiology textbook *Exercise Physiology: Nutrition, Energy, and Human Performance*:

> "A carbohydrate deficient diet rapidly depletes muscle and liver glycogen and negatively affects performance in short term, anaerobic exercise, and prolonged high-intensity aerobic activities. These observations relate particularly to individuals who modify their diets by reducing carbohydrate intake below recommended levels. Reliance on starvation diets or other potentially harmful diets (e.g., high-fat, low-carbohydrate diets, "liquid protein" diets, or water diets), proves counterproductive for weight control, exercise performance, optimal nutrition, and good health. Low-carbohydrate diets make it difficult from an energy supply standpoint to participate regularly in vigorous, longer duration physical activities."[311]

---

309 Asker E. Jeukendrup. High-carbohydrate versus high-fat diets in endurance sports.

310 http://www.ncbi.nlm.nih.gov/pubmed/17617997

311 Exercise Physiology: Nutrition, Energy, and Human Performance

Another comprehensive review on the performance effects of fat-adaptation titled "Adaptation to a fat-rich diet: effects on endurance performance in humans" concluded:

> **"When adaptation to a fat-rich diet was performed over longer periods, studies where performance was tested at moderate intensity, 60 to 80% of maximal oxygen uptake, demonstrate either no difference or an attenuated performance after consumption of a fat-rich compared with a carbohydrate-rich diet. When performance was measured at high intensity after a longer period of adaptation, it was at best maintained, but in most cases attenuated, compared with consuming a carbohydrate-rich diet."**[312]

According to Phinney himself—the researcher often cited by low-carb advocates—assuming one pays very "careful attention" to "keto adaptation, mineral nutriture, and constraint of the daily protein dose" along with strict carbohydrate restriction, one can, at best, *maintain* one's aerobic endurance performance roughly as well as one performs on a diet with ample dietary carbohydrates. He concludes that "therapeutic use of ketogenic diets should not require constraint of most forms of physical labor or recreational activity, with the one caveat that anaerobic (i.e., weight lifting or sprint) performance is limited by the low muscle glycogen levels induced by a ketogenic diet, and **this would strongly discourage its use under most conditions of competitive athletics."**[313]

Does this sound like a secret magical fuel source that powers superhuman performance?

Or does it sound like a lot of effort, time, and dietary deprivation to achieve basically nothing except the same aerobic performance (assuming you do everything correctly) and a guaranteed decline in performance in anything that requires high-intensity bursts (i.e., most sports)?

---

312 http://www.ncbi.nlm.nih.gov/pubmed/11103848

313 http://www.ncbi.nlm.nih.gov/pmc/articles/PMC524027/

SUMMARY

The take-home message is that training in a ketogenic or near ketogenic state has no clear value in improving athletic performance. For endurance athletes, at best they can hope to *maintain* their performance or perhaps be one of the lucky anomalies who seem to increase their performance. **Most athletes in non-endurance sports (most sports) can expect significant declines in their performance—roughly in proportion to their sport's demands for bursts of high-intensity activity.**

So why do low-carb advocates push this way of eating, with such sparse supportive evidence? We are unaware of any coaches or exercise physiologists working with national or professional sports teams or long-term, high-level, elite sport performers who advocate low-carb eating and competing on ketogenic diets. And where athletes do exist who are attempting to follow low-carb diets, there is little evidence that such practices have improved their performance.

Once you get past all the hype from the low-carb advocates (who are intent on conducting study after study *trying* so very hard to show that carbohydrate restriction leads to any sort of performance benefit), you find the simple scientific reality that performance benefits of low-carb diets are *minimal at best,* and, at worst, one sees a substantial decline in performance. The studies bear out this conclusion over and over again.

Thus the question is, if the science shows such minimal and unpredictable benefits along with a strong potential for a dramatic *reduction* in performance, what is the point?

For an athlete, the answer is that there is no point in doing any diet unless the diet change is *proven* to reliably improve performance and well-being. Virtually all scientific studies to date and the evolved practices of elite athletes (and their coaches) point to the superiority of a moderate to high carbohydrate intake over low-carb/ketogenic diets for performance.

The reason that low-carb, high-fat diets aren't popular in high-level athletics is *not* because all the scientists conducting research in these fields for the last several decades are ignorant of the "wonders" of fat-adaptation, or that such diets haven't yet been scientifically tested. To the contrary, the notion that fat-adaptation could lead to enhanced athletic performance has

been around for a long time, and it has been tested extensively. The reason virtually no elite athletes in any sport use it is that it has been found *not* to provide performance benefit in most cases, and much of the time, it has been found to significantly *decrease* performance.

Chapter 6: The "Fat Burning" Scam

There are thousands of people out there trying to sell you on the low-carb "fat-burning" diet mythology. There are all sorts of claims that have been made by low-carb gurus about how being a "fat burner" rather than a "carb burner" results in all sorts of miraculous effects on health, energy level, athletic performance, longevity, and fat loss.

This mythology revolves around a few things:

- The notion that our ancestors ate a low-carb diet—as many modern-day Paleo diet advocates claim.
- The claim that the body's "preferred" fuel source is fat, not carbohydrates. (This is largely based on the claim that our ancestors ate low-carb diets.)
- The idea that carbohydrates are not "essential" nutrients like certain fatty acids and certain amino acids have been labeled "essential." And since they are not "essential," they are therefore less important than fats and proteins.
- The claim that eating carbohydrates causes energy spikes and "crashes" and that fat is a better fuel source because it provides "steady energy."
- That being in a state of fat burning (and/or ketosis) is a "metabolically advantaged" state that confers health and/or performance benefits.

- Most important, the general misunderstanding and confusion around the difference between being a "fat burner" and actually burning *body fat.*

Did Our Ancestors Eat Low-Carb Diets?

One of the foundational premises of the low-carb Paleo movement has been that our Paleolithic ancestors—hunter-gatherer humans—ate a low-carb diet. It is typically stated by low-carb gurus as something like what Mark Sisson, author of *The Primal Blueprint*, says here:

"Fat and protein were the dominant macronutrients (when food was even available) over the majority of our two-and-a-half million years as evolving humans. The lack of regular access to food and a scarcity of carbohydrates for much of this time necessitated that we adapt efficient pathways to readily store and access body fat for energy if we were to survive day-to-day and generation-to-generation. Our movement patterns were such that we never required large amounts of glucose or that we needed to store very much glycogen. **It was predominantly fats, ketones, and the minimal infusion of glucose via gluconeogenesis that got us here. Dietary carbs were insignificant.**"[314]

It's an interesting idea, but one that is based far more on speculation and wishful thinking than science.

The truth is that we do not need to invoke speculative theories about what our ancestors ate hundreds of thousands of years ago—we can simply look at traditional peoples that exist in the world today that are still eating the same diet they've been eating for thousands of years and look at what they eat every day.

As it turns out, there is a huge variance in the diet of traditional populations around the world today.

Some—like the Inuit, and the Sami of Scandinavia—eat low-carbohydrate diets of almost entirely animal protein and fat, and berries whenever the weather is warm enough. Others—like the Hiwi and Ache tribes of South America, the Onge of the Andaman Islands, and the Anbarra of Australia—eat animal food-based diets that also include ample carbohydrates from tubers and/or fruits and/or honey. Countless other traditional populations—like the Tukisenta, the Kitavans, the !Kung, the Hadza, the Ewe tribe, the Kuna of Panama, the Okinawans, and most of the entire continent of Asia—have existed on carbohydrate-based diets for hundreds or thousands of years.

---

314 http://www.marksdailyapple.com/a-metabolic-paradigm-shift-fat-carbs-human-body-metabolism/

In addition, we have good anthropological evidence suggesting that carbohydrate-rich foods have been a large part of the human diet for many thousands of years:

- Research published in the journal *Nature* reports that the majority of the diet of our very early human ancestors was similar to that of chimpanzees—mostly consisting of leaves, fruits, wood, and bark.[315]
- Another study found that people living in what is now Mozambique, along the eastern coast of Africa, likely ate a diet rich in the grain sorghum as far back as 105,000 years ago.[316]
- Research presented in a 2011 issue of *Proceedings of the National Academy of Science* showed that remnants of starchy grains have been found on the teeth of Neanderthal skeletons all over Europe and the Middle East.[317]
- A 2010 issue of the *Proceedings of the National Academy of Science* suggested that eating starchy grains from wild plants (and perhaps grinding them into flour) was a widespread practice in Europe during the Paleolithic period.[318]

So it is scientifically misguided to make sweeping generalizations like "our ancestors ate low-carb" or "fat and protein were the dominant macronutrients over the majority of our two-and-a-half million years as evolving humans." These claims are simply false.

No such generalizations about the macronutrient content of the diet of "our ancestors" can be made. And if one is so inclined, one could just as easily make the case—based on which populations one selects—that, in fact, our ancestors ate predominately carbohydrate-based diets.

But such sweeping generalizations are anathema to good science.

The truth is that no such broad statements can be made about "our ancestors' diet" because our ancestors' diets ranged from near-complete carnivory to near-complete vegetarianism, and everything in between.

---

315 http://www.nytimes.com/2012/06/28/science/australopithecus-sediba-preferred-forest-foods-fossil-teeth-suggest.html?_r=0

316 http://www.ncbi.nlm.nih.gov/pubmed/20019285

317 http://www.ncbi.nlm.nih.gov/pubmed/21187393

318 http://www.ncbi.nlm.nih.gov/pubmed/21187393

A Breakdown of Different Traditional Diets

LOW-CARB POPULATIONS:

The Inuit and the Sami tribes are examples of low-carb populations. They live in Arctic and subarctic regions where plant food is relatively scarce—particularly in winter months.

Sami

The Sami are primarily hunters and fishers (they also herd reindeer), with some plant use. Animals used for food include reindeer, moose, bear, seals, walrus, salmon, and rabbits. Carbohydrate-containing plant foods primarily consist of various berries like blueberries, cloudberries, lingonberries, and others, which they get whenever they are available.[319]

Inuit

The Inuit rely primarily on animal foods including seals, walrus, caribou, fish, shellfish, and other marine animals, and a relatively small amount of plant foods including root vegetables and berries, as well as some partially digested plant matter (lichens, assorted grasses) found in hunted caribou stomachs. [320]

Note that even while relying almost exclusively on a diet of animal flesh and blubber, the Inuit STILL eat carbohydrates (upwards of 50g per day) in the form of stored glycogen in the meat of the animals they eat.

Both of these tribes are fairly low-carb with about 35% of the diet coming from protein, 50% from fat, and 15-20% from carbohydrates. This is as low carb as it gets in the wild. Yet, this diet is certainly not devoid of carbohydrates, and as Richard Nikoley noted on his blog, even these cultures made an effort to obtain carbohydrates from berries, nuts, seaweed, and tubers whenever they could.[321]

---

319 The Cambridge Encyclopedia of Hunters and Gatherers [Richard B. Lee, Richard Daly]

320 The Cambridge Encyclopedia of Hunters and Gatherers [Richard B. Lee, Richard Daly]

321 http://freetheanimal.com/2014/03/disrupting-carbs-prebiotics.html

MODERATE-CARB POPULATIONS:

These populations consume ample animal foods but eat considerably more plants and carbohydrate-containing foods than the Sami or Inuit.

Hiwi

The Hiwi live in western Venezuela and eastern Colombia, where they consume a diet of hunted game (such as deer, capybara, armadillo, caiman, turtles, and lizards), fish, gathered roots, and some honey. [322]

Ache

The Ache live in the tropical forests of eastern Paraguay where they eat a diet of hunted game (armadillo, deer, capuchin monkey, etc.), honey, palm starch, and insect larvae.[323]

!Kung

The !Kung tribe live in the Kalahari Desert of Africa where they consume a diet of primarily mongongo nuts (a nut rich in both fat and carbs), baobob fruit, berries, wild mangos, roots/tubers, and wild game (antelope, rabbit, guinea fowl, and giraffe).[324]

Anbarra

The Anbarra live on the coast of Northern Australia and eat a diet of largely shellfish and other marine animals, with ample root vegetables, fruits, and seeds. [325]

---

322 The Cambridge Encyclopedia of Hunters and Gatherers [Richard B. Lee, Richard Daly]

323 The Cambridge Encyclopedia of Hunters and Gatherers [Richard B. Lee, Richard Daly]

324 http://anthropology.ua.edu/bindon/ant476/topics/Foragers.pdf

325 The Cambridge Encyclopedia of Hunters and Gatherers [Richard B. Lee, Richard Daly]

Onge

The Onge tribe lives in the Andaman Islands south of India and consume a diet of wild game (wild boar, turtles, fish, crabs, dugongs), as well as root vegetables, fruit, and honey. [326]

HIGH-CARB POPULATIONS:

Hadza

The Hadza tribe lives in Tanzania, where they eat a plant-based diet of mostly tubers, berries, honey, baobob fruit, and some very lean wild game (birds and some mammals). [327]

Tukisenta

The Tukisenta tribe in New Guinea eats an almost entirely pure carbohydrate diet composed of starchy tubers.[328]

West Nile district in Uganda

This population was studied during the 1940s and was eating a carbohydrate-rich diet consisting mainly of cassava, bananas, millet, corn, lentils, peanuts, and vegetables. [329]

Nearly the entire continent of Asia during the 20th century

Millions of people on the entire continent of Asia have been eating a carbohydrate-heavy, plant-based diet for thousands of years. It is largely based on white rice, as well as root vegetables, along with some fruit. [330]

Pima Indians

---

326 The Cambridge Encyclopedia of Hunters and Gatherers [Richard B. Lee, Richard Daly]

327 http://wholehealthsource.blogspot.com/2012/06/sugar-intake-and-body-fatness-in-non.html

328 http://wholehealthsource.blogspot.com/2011/08/carbohydrate-hypothesis-of-obesity.html

329 http://wholehealthsource.blogspot.com/2011/08/carbohydrate-hypothesis-of-obesity.html

330 http://wholehealthsource.blogspot.com/2011/08/carbohydrate-hypothesis-of-obesity.html

The Pima Indians are a very famous group within the obesity research community, largely because obesity rates are so incredibly high. Their traditional diet was roughly 70% carbohydrate. As explained previously, they became obese in conjunction with a progressive lowering of carbohydrate content of the diet and an increase in the fat content. [331]

Tarahumara Indians of Mexico

This group eats a traditional diet of mostly corn, beans, rice, and squash, and has an extremely low incidence of type II diabetes. Their diet is 12% fat and over 75% carbohydrate.[332]

Kitavans

The Kitavans, as the name implies, live on the South Pacific island of Kitava. Dr. Staffan Lindeberg researched this population heavily during the 1990s and found that their diet consisted mostly of taro, sweet potatoes, cassava, fruit, coconut, and seafood. They ate about 50g a day of unrefined sugar from fruit. Their diet came in at a whopping 69% carbohydrate. [333]

Ewe tribe

The Ewe tribe in Togo, Africa, eats a diet composed almost entirely of starchy tubers. [334]

Kuna

The Kuna population off the coast of Panama eats a carbohydrate-based diet that is centered around plantains, corn, cassava, kidney beans, coconuts, a variety of fruits, chocolate, and some wild game and seafood. (Interestingly, they are lean despite also having some modern junk food in their diet such as Kool-Aid, doughnuts, and pure sugar

---

331 http://wholehealthsource.blogspot.com/2008/05/lessons-from-pima-indians.html Guyenet, S. (2008, May 15). Lessons from the Pima Indians. Retrieved from http://wholehealthsource.blogspot.com/2008/05/lessons-from-pima-indians.html.

332 http://ajcn.nutrition.org/content/32/4/905.full.pdf

333 http://wholehealthsource.blogspot.com/2008/08/kitavans-wisdom-from-pacific-islands.html

334 http://www.weightymatters.ca/2012/09/the-ewe-super-high-carb-diet-992.html

added to a cocoa beverage consumed daily, in addition to all the other carbohydrate-rich staple foods they consume daily.)[335]

The most thorough information ever complied on diets of humans still living in traditional ways comes from Staffan Lindeberg's *Food and Western Disease*. This is perhaps the only *real* "Paleo" book ever written. Here are some relevant quotes from Lindeberg's book regarding the diet of our ancestors.[336]

> "What did humans eat in their original environment? A simple answer is: Food that was available and that provided dietary energy with a reasonable amount of effort, such as fruits, vegetables, nuts, insects, larvae, wild game meat, fish, shellfish, and root vegetables. However, it is difficult to define what we mean by 'original,' since most of the shaping of human digestion and metabolism took place long before we became human-like and started to walk on two legs, approximately 6 million years ago. Hence, it could be argued that the Miocene vegetarian-like habitats, from 23 to 5 million years ago, provide a proper reference for human nutrition. In contrast, others argue that later habitats exerted such strong selection pressures that humans became adapted to a high intake of meat. However, neither position excludes the other. We may be adapted to any kind of food without necessarily being dependent on it for high reproductive success."
>
> "Furthermore, archaeological reconstructions of past diets from morphological characteristics of bones and teeth, analyses of remaining tools, and measurements of bone chemistry do not provide strong evidence in a particular direction, except that we were omnivores."
>
> **"Our primate ancestors probably consumed large amounts of fruit regularly during 50 million years until they became bipedal around 6 million years ago. Today, fruit makes up more than 75% of the diet for chimpanzees, bonobos, and orangutans. ... Human preference for sweet food clearly suggests that our ancestors would have savored one**

---

335 http://wholehealthsource.blogspot.com/2008/03/say-hello-to-kuna.html

336 Lindeberg, S. Food and Western Disease

> **exquisite choice: honey.** It may have been a major source of concentrated sweetness, and for several contemporary hunter-gatherers the intake has been considerable during the honey season."
>
> "Increasing evidence suggests that large starchy underground storage organs (roots, tubers, bulbs, and corms), which plants form in dry climates, were staple foods 1–2 million years ago."
>
> "The excellent health status among this and other starch-eating ethnic groups, including our own study population in Papua New Guinea, contradicts the popular notion that such foods are a cause of obesity and type 2 diabetes."
>
> "Even the most dedicated meat eaters in ancient times most probably had an intake of healthy plant foods that sharply exceeded that of most modern humans."
>
> "In most habitats, the consumption of insects and larvae may have been substantial and would have provided an important source of protein and fat. Western society has long resisted such food, but other cultures in the world often value them highly, and they are regularly consumed by non-human primates."
>
> "To summarize the evidence from different fields of science, **humans are apparently omnivores who are well adapted for a diet based either on animal or plant foods, the relative proportions of which have been highly variable depending on habitat.** The discussion about human's ancient diets is often misdirected to a debate on meat versus plant foods. Thereby, the main point is missed: most of the calories in Western countries are provided by foods that were practically unavailable during human evolution."

The simple fact is that there is no evidence whatsoever that low-carb nutrition was standard fare for our cavemen ancestors. This theory is romantically oversimplified and wrong.

To the contrary, there is overwhelming evidence that carbohydrates—mainly from root vegetables, tubers, fruits, grains, and even concentrated sugar in the form of honey—have formed the foundation of the diet of countless non-industrialized humans for tens of thousands of years.

In fact, for thousands of years, dozens of hunter-gatherer tribes all over the world have gone to great lengths—while risking painful bee stings among other dangers—to smoke out bees from their hive and run off with their honey. The Rai people of Nepal scale huge cliffs and perch themselves on shaky ladders to harvest their honey. The Hadza of Africa consume about 15% of their calories from honey. The Aranda tribe of Australia, the Batek of Malaysia, the Yanomami of Venezuela, the Shenko Honeymen of Ethiopia, the Aka, Mbuti, and Efe tribes of the Congo, and the Ache of Paraguay—all of these tribes consume a significant portion of their diet from honey.[337] [338] **The Mbuti consumes a whopping 80% of their total daily calories from honey during the rainy season, and members of the Ache tribe sometimes consume over 1,000 calories a day from pure honey!**[339] [340] So it's not as if consuming large amounts of sugar is foreign to the human species.

Anyone who makes blanket generalizations like "our Paleolithic ancestors ate low-carb and were fat burners" (as many popular Paleo gurus claim), or the opposite claim that "our Paleolithic ancestors ate an entirely plant-foods diet" (as many vegetarian gurus claim), is someone not worth listening to because they either haven't done enough research or they are deliberately ignoring evidence that counters their dietary ideology.

Commonly, we see people of various dietary dogmas cherry-picking the diets of various tribes in order to give validation to their particular dogmas. By cherry-picking the research and then listing off various Arctic tribes, one can easily give the impression that "all our ancestors ate low-carb." One could also easily exclude the Arctic peoples and look at the vast majority of non-Arctic peoples and find that many of those populations ate a carbohydrate-rich diet, and say, "all our ancestors ate carbohydrate-based diets."

---

337 http://freetheanimal.com/2015/01/hormesis-afraid-unrefined.html

338 http://www.smithsonianmag.com/science-nature/humans-the-honey-hunters-9760262/?no-ist

339 http://jambo.africa.kyoto-u.ac.jp/kiroku/asm_normal/abstracts/pdf/ASM%20%20Vol.1%201981/Mitsuo%20ICHIKAWA.pdf

340 http://www.smithsonianmag.com/science-nature/humans-the-honey-hunters-9760262/

The truth is that the diets of our Paleolithic ancestors varied wildly in terms of macronutrients. Data from indigenous cultures around the world has shown it to be possible for humans to survive with good longevity on widely ranging diets, from near-vegetarian diets based solely on plant foods like legumes and vegetables, to the meat, blood, and dairy diet of the Maasai, to nearly pure carbohydrate diets of the Tukisenta and Ewe peoples, to the almost complete animal flesh diet of some Arctic tribes, to the rice-based diet of much of Asia.

If we try to find any indications of which one of these is healthier—for example, if we compare Arctic peoples who eat mostly animal foods with rice-eating Asians or the Tukisenta and Ewe who basically eat nothing but carbohydrates from sweet potatoes, we do not see a clear picture emerge regarding one of these being superior in terms of body composition or lifespan or rates of degenerative disease.

Some low-carb advocates have tried to paint a picture that certain low-carb, high-fat diet eating tribes are of robust health and are free from degenerative diseases like heart disease, for example, the notion that the Inuit or Maasai peoples are free of heart disease despite consuming very high amounts of fat. Yet, these claims appear to be based on lack of good studies on the subject more than anything. A 2014 study published in the *Canadian Journal of Cardiology* showed that cardiovascular disease has been at least as frequent among northern native populations like the Inuit as for neighboring populations consuming a more typical Western diet.[341] Strokes are also not uncommon. Overall life expectancy was found to be about a decade shorter. Heart disease seemed rare among northern native populations mainly because reporting of medical problems is not consistent. It is also claimed that the Maasai people are free of heart disease despite consuming their high-fat diet, yet, one researcher who has actually studies the hearts of deceased Maasai stated, "We have collected hearts and aortae from 50 authenticated Maasai men who died of trauma and we found extensive atherosclerosis."[342] So this notion that many of the

341 http://www.onlinecjc.ca/article/S0828-282X(14)00237-2/abstract

342 Mann GV. The Masai, milk, and the yogurt factor: an alternative explanation. Atherosclerosis. 1978;29:265.

tribes eating low-carb, high-fat diets are free of disease and have exceptional health has little basis in science.

But long-term randomized controlled trials comparing the longevity or incidence of heart disease on these different diets simply have not been done. It may eventually turn out that it is possible to have health and longevity on low-carb, high-fat diets as good as many of the known long-lived populations that consume higher carbohydrate diets lower in fat, but there is currently little evidence—either from long-term RCTs or from epidemiological evidence—to suggest that such diets are as good or are in any way superior for disease prevention or longevity.

Simply put, there isn't any macronutrient composition of the diet that is "the diet of our ancestors." Nor is there clear evidence that health and longevity are strongly linked with macronutrient composition of the diet. Summarizing the data on the traditional human diet, Guyenet states, "Like all other animals, humans are healthy and robust when occupying their preferred ecological niche. Our niche happens to be a particularly broad one, ranging from near-complete carnivory to plant-rich omnivory. But it does not include large amounts of industrial foods." [343]

If we were to try to form a generalized picture of the diet of our ancestors, it might look something like this:

- It is an omnivorous diet with a mix of plant and animal foods.
- It is a whole-foods diet, not a diet with significant quantities of refined industrial foods.
- In Arctic climates where plants don't grow particularly well, tribes rely on a large portion of the diet from animal foods.
- In non-Arctic climates—where the vast majority of humans have lived historically—most tribes have subsisted on diets with a large portion of overall calories from carbohydrate-rich plant foods. These diets may rely heavily on animal foods in addition to those carbohydrates, or they may rely almost exclusively on the carbohydrate-rich plant foods. Most of these populations ate starchy root vegetables and tubers, or in some cases, rice, corn, or ancient grains like sorghum and teff. It is also common

343 http://wholehealthsource.blogspot.com/2008/08/kitavans-wisdom-from-pacific-islands.html

for traditional people to eat sugar-rich foods like fruit and honey.

There is no indication that populations eating large amounts of carbohydrates have *any deleterious* health or body composition issues relative to low-carb, high-fat eating populations. There is no tremendous improvement in health or body composition that one finds when examining the low-carb, high-fat eating Inuit relative to the high-carb eating Kitavans. Or the Sami relative to the Hadza. Or the Maasai relative to the Tukisenta.

Moreover, most of our ancestors were seeking calories to survive environments that were far less abundant in food than the modern environment. So it makes no sense that they would pass on more readily available fruit and tubers in favor of low-calorie leafy greens or Paleolithic versions of cauliflower.

That leaves us with a curious thought: **How did the Paleo movement—a philosophy that is based on the premise that we should live in a way that is in harmony with our ancestors' lifestyle—get hijacked by this low-carb nonsense that humans are only supposed to eat low-carb diets, when the science provides ample evidence that these anti-carb recommendations are incongruent with the diets of countless hunter-gatherer and traditional peoples?**

Going "Paleo" doesn't require speculative unscientific and nonsensical theories regarding how our hunter-gatherer ancestors ate and lived. We can simply look to modern-day, non-Westernized tribal populations and hunter-gatherers to see that a whole-food diet based on a foundation of ample unrefined carbohydrates—mainly root vegetables and/or fruits—is at least as congruent with our genetic makeup and physiology as meat and animal fat.

Based on an analysis of past and contemporary hunter-gatherers, there is simply no scientific basis whatsoever to suggest that a low-carbohydrate diet was the diet of our Paleolithic ancestors, or that it is the optimal diet for which our genes are designed.

What is the Body's Preferred Source of Fuel—Fat or Carbohydrates?

First, let's address the foundational assertion that underlies all the these various claims that wiring the body to be more of a "fat burner" has some panacea-like effect—the notion that fats (not carbs) are the preferred source of fuel by the body.

The typical way that this is presented by low-carb gurus is that our bodies are wired to run off fats—not carbs—for fuel (since our ancestors, according to them, ate low-carb diets of mostly animal foods, nuts/seeds, and green leafy vegetables), and thus, running on fats is the way evolution has designed our bodies to run. Here's Mark Sisson, author of *The Primal Blueprint,* on the matter:

"The truth is, fat is the preferred fuel of human metabolism and has been for most of human evolution. Under normal human circumstances, we actually require only minimal amounts of glucose, most or all of which can be supplied by the liver as needed on a daily basis. The simple SAD fact that carbs/glucose are so readily available and cheap today doesn't mean that we should depend on them as a primary source of fuel or revere them so highly. In fact, it is this blind allegiance to the 'Carb Paradigm' that has driven so many of us to experience the vast array of metabolic problems that threaten to overwhelm our health care system. … It follows logically that if you can limit carb intake to a range of which is absolutely necessary [Note: This 'absolutely necessary' amount is apparently less than 100g per day, according to Sisson] and make the difference up with tasty fats and protein, you can literally reprogram your genes back to the evolutionary-based factory setting you had at birth—the setting that offered you the opportunity to start life as a truly efficient fat-burning organism and to continue to do so for the rest of your life as long as you send the right signals to your genes. Becoming an efficient fat burner is the major premise of the Primal Blueprint eating and exercise strategies."[344]

Now, as we have already shown you, essentially every single one of these statements is false. Fat and protein are not the dominant macronutrients for anyone but those living in Arctic environments

344 http://www.marksdailyapple.com/a-metabolic-paradigm-shift-fat-carbs-human-body-metabolism/#axzz3JpQUwEiJ

where plants don't grow. Pretty much every other population in every part of the world that still lives their traditional lifestyle eats carbohydrate-based diets or, at the very least, consumes ample carbohydrates daily. Numerous tribes in Africa and Asia consume diets of essentially nothing but carbohydrates. **So these fantasies of our ancestors "eating nothing but protein and fat" are completely unscientific and polar opposite of the reality for numerous traditional populations around the world that have been studied and had their diet composition analyzed.**

Another variation on this theme that fat is the "preferred fuel" of the body is the ketogenic trend in the low-carb community. These people go to great lengths to avoid even very small amounts of carbohydrates, while taking in huge quantities of fat, in order to coax their body into a state of ketosis (where it is using ketone bodies as a major fuel source). This state, they claim, is the "default physiological state" of the body.

There's just one problem with this theory: **there is not a single population on the planet that appears to operate in a state of ketosis.**

Even in populations that eat a diet of almost entirely animal foods like the Inuit—who most people would think are eating a diet of purely protein and fat—the fact is that in fresh meat, there is a fairly large quantity of carbohydrates in the form of glycogen stored in the muscle tissue. For example, it was found that even in the Inuit, they were consuming well over 50g of carbohydrates per day just from eating meat! This was enough to keep them out of nutritional ketosis, and when scientists checked their bodies for ketones, only very low (normal) levels were found.[345] (Note that a higher protein intake will also knock a person out of ketosis, so this may be another reason why the Inuit are not in ketosis.)

This was rather shocking to the low-carb Paleo advocates who try to suggest that ketosis is the default physiological state of our hunter-gatherer ancestors. The fact is that even among people who have virtually no access to plant foods and eat a diet almost entirely of blubber-rich animal foods, they *still* consume enough carbohydrates and protein to stay out of nutritional ketosis.

---

345 http://freetheanimal.com/2014/03/reiterate-elevated-ketone.html

Moreover, getting into nutritional ketosis requires both a low-carbohydrate and *low-protein* diet. In other words, getting into this state requires you to deprive your body of *two* of the three macronutrients and feed it mainly a diet of fat. (It's also worth noting that it is virtually impossible to achieve this level of fat in the diet without consuming processed foods [e.g. refined oils] or discarding part of the whole food.) Either a decent amount of carbohydrates or protein will kick the body out of ketosis.

Logically, it makes absolutely no sense to say that our "default" physiological state requires us to systematically deprive the body of two of the three macronutrients.

Moreover, the body's preferred physiological state is the one the body operates in when it has a *choice* of which state to operate in—that is, when it is provided numerous options for fuel. When provided with ample carbohydrates or protein, the body does not operate in ketosis. It doesn't even operate in ketosis in the Inuit people who eat a diet of virtually all animal foods with huge amounts of fat!

Now, this is not to say that ketosis is inherently "bad" or something of that nature. In fact, occasional bouts of ketosis (in the context of intermittent fasting) may indeed have profound health benefits. And ketosis also clearly has value in treating certain conditions (neurological disease, epilepsy, etc.).

But it is clear that ketones are not some mystical and secret fuel source that confers amazing benefits for health or performance to those without these specific diseases (i.e., the vast majority of people).

Also clear is that ketosis is *not* the "preferred" metabolic state of the body.

If ketosis were a default or "preferred" state of physiology, then:

1) **There would be numerous examples of traditional populations who can be verified to be in ketosis. (There aren't.)**
2) **The body would operate in ketosis regardless of which nutrients were available to it. (It doesn't.)**
3) **The body would not slip out of ketosis so easily. (It does.)**

So what is our "preferred" fuel source?

The simple fact is that there is no such talk of any "preferred" fuel in biochemistry or physiology textbooks. This is largely a made-up notion.

But just to play along with this debate of our "preferred" fuel source, consider the simple fact that if given the choice between burning carbohydrates or fat, our cells preferentially use carbohydrates for fuel.

Take a close look at this quote from obesity researcher Stephan Guyenet:

> **"When a diet of mixed macronutrient composition is eaten to excess, the carbohydrate is preferentially burned off, while the fat is mostly shunted into fat tissue.** This makes sense because why would the body go through the inefficient process of converting carbohydrate to fat for storage when it can just shunt dietary fat directly into fat tissue?"

Pay particular attention to the first part of that quote—the part about when you eat a diet of both fat and carbohydrates, the body *preferentially* uses carbohydrates for fuel.

Now, let's look at another quote from a physiology expert, Lyle McDonald, author of *The Ketogenic Diet*:

> **"So what happens when you provide the body with both carbs and fats in the diet? Which fuel source is preferred? Well the answer is clear: carbs. That is, when you give the body both carbs and fats (or more generally when carbs are available), the body will use the carbs for fuel and store the fat ... if the body is given a choice of carbs or fats, it will prefer carbs for fuel. No question and no debates."**[346]

So if you have appreciation for the intelligence of the body from millions of years of evolution—for example, if you are inclined towards a more naturalistic or Paleo philosophy--this simple fact shows us that if anything is our "preferred" fuel source, it's carbohydrates.

By the way, the body's preferred choice of carbohydrates over fat for fuel is the most pronounced in young, healthy, lean people, and

346 http://www.bodyrecomposition.com/fat-loss/is-fat-preferred-fuel-source-body-qa.html

especially athletes of high-intensity sports like sprinting (you know, the people with the leanest, most beautiful bodies on the planet). The younger, healthier, and leaner you are, and the more high-intensity sports you do, the more your body will prefer to use carbohydrates as its dominant fuel source. The more fat, unhealthy, sedentary, insulin resistant (diabetic), and old you are, the harder time your body has in accessing and burning carbohydrates efficiently, and the more you become a fat burner.

Again, the simple fact to pay attention to is this: if you take a young healthy person and feed them a diet with ample carbohydrates and ample fat, their body will predominantly use carbohydrates for fuel. If given the choice, the human body will always choose to use carbs rather than fat for fuel. And the only way it becomes possible for your body to use fats as the dominant fuel source is by forcibly depriving it of its preferred fuel source (carbohydrates). In other words, the whole idea of the low-carb gurus that your body "prefers" to use fat for fuel, or that it is better for performance or healthier to use fat for fuel, is complete rubbish.

The fat-burning fantasy is based on a fundamentally foolish assumption that the human body is stupid, doesn't know what's good for it, and *requires you to forcibly deprive your body of a certain nutrient so it can operate in its supposedly "preferred" way of being.*

Does that sound idiotic to you? It should.

So unless you're going to suggest that millions of years of evolution have programmed the human body in such a way that the body is stupid and doesn't know what's good for it, then it is clear that carbs are the body's preferred fuel source for optimal cellular function.

Now, having said that, this isn't all black and white. For example, the preferred fuel source of the heart muscle is indeed fats! And most of the cells of the body run on a mix of both sugar and fat throughout the day. It is clear that the body *does* prefer to use *both* fuel sources, pretty much all the time. Young healthy bodies generally have the ability to shift back and forth between fuel sources with ease—depending upon activity needs and the fuel sources being provided in the diet (something called metabolic flexibility), while metabolically unhealthy people generally lose this capacity to some extent. The truth isn't a black-and-white extreme of "carbs are great and fats are the devil." Both are very good fuel sources, and the body likes to run on a mix of both of them.

But, it is very clear that fats are *not* some undiscovered secret fuel source with amazing benefits. If given the choice of what fuel to run on, carbs are clearly the preferred fuel source of the body. That simple fact should tell you most of what you need to know.

The Myth that Carbohydrates Are Not "Essential"

Get ready to enter the twilight zone of nutrition—the realm of completely twisted and, to be blunt, rather silly logic from low-carb advocates.

Many low-carb Paleo diet advocates try to assert the superiority of fat as a fuel for the body by saying "there is no such thing as an 'essential' carbohydrate."

What they mean by this is that we have "essential" amino acids and "essential" fatty acids—that is, proteins and fats that must be included in the diet for you to stay alive—yet, with carbohydrates, the body can stay alive without any carbohydrates in the diet whatsoever. Therefore, this logic goes, because our bodies can live and breathe while on a zero-carb diet eating nothing but protein and fat, that means that protein and fat are really vital for your cells to function, but carbohydrates are not.

Their logic seems to make sense, right? If the body can stay alive without you eating any carbohydrates, it must mean that carbohydrates aren't that important, right? The body can take them or leave them—so to speak—so, they mustn't be all that crucial for cell function, right?

Well, except that upon closer inspection, we see some giant holes appear that show just how foolish this argument really is:

1) Low-carb gurus typically advise people to consume the *majority* of their daily calories from saturated and monounsaturated fats. They also go to great lengths to convince us that dietary cholesterol is healthy and we should eat it in abundance because it so vital to our cellular health. Ironically, the body also has *no dietary requirement* for saturated fats, monounsaturated fats, or dietary cholesterol. That is, these nutrients are *also* not "essential" since the body can live without them in exactly the same way it can live without carbohydrates. Thus, these low-carb gurus are suggesting that carbs aren't important on the basis that they aren't "essential" and then simultaneously recommending that you eat the majority of your daily calories from other nutrients that are also not "essential." On what planet does this make any sense?
2) They often build this notion of how unimportant carbohydrates are around the idea that "there's only one teaspoon of sugar

floating around in the blood," as if to say that this seemingly meager amount of sugar in the blood at any given time suggests that sugar can't possibly be that important. How could we need lots of carbs every day if we only have the seemingly tiny amount of five grams floating around in our bloodstream? Makes sense, right? Surely, carbohydrates aren't important if there's only a measly five grams in the bloodstream. The only problem with this logic is that we have *even fewer* fatty acids (the fuel source they claim is so much more "essential" than carbohydrates) floating around in our blood at any given time. But they like to conveniently leave that part out. If sugar is unimportant based on the fact that "only five grams are present in the blood at any given time," then how is it that fats are so important when there's only one-fifth to one-tenth of that amount of non-esterified fatty acids (the kind used in fat burning) in the blood at any given time?[347]

3) It is indeed true that the body can stay alive in the absence of dietary carbohydrates. However, this is *not* due to the body entering a state of physiology where it is no longer relying on carbohydrates for fuel. (If that were the case, it would indeed lend credence to the idea that carbohydrates aren't important to our cells.) **Rather, it is because our bodies are designed to *still* be able to run on carbohydrates—even when none are being consumed in the diet!**

No doubt you've heard the term "blood sugar" before, right? Let's think about that for a moment—"blood sugar" means that there's a bunch of sugar molecules floating around in your blood. I can hear the low-carb dieters now saying to themselves, "Oooh, but I thought sugar is toxic—I don't want any of that icky stuff floating around in my blood!" Well, like it or not, you have a bunch of sugar molecules—millions of them actually—floating around in your blood all the time, day and night, whether you're awake or asleep. So this leads us to a somewhat obvious question that is almost universally ignored by advocates of low-carb diets: Why do our bodies have blood sugar? You know, if sugar is evil toxic stuff, and if our cells prefer to run on fat, why exactly do we have sugar floating around in our blood at a

347 http://carbsanity.blogspot.com/2012/06/theres-no-dietary-need-for-saturated.html

constant level all the time—even when eating no carbohydrates in the diet? Why, in fact, are our bodies almost always running mechanisms to produce new sugars (gluconeogenesis) and keep sugar levels constant in the blood?

Simple: **Because our cells are constantly *taking in and using* that sugar as fuel to make the cellular energy that keeps your cells alive.**

In fact, your cells love using sugar for fuel so much that even when you're eating a near *zero*-carbohydrate diet, your body *still* maintains the proper level of sugar floating around in the blood. Yes, you can be eating virtually no carbohydrates at all in your diet for multiple days, yet you will still have millions of sugar molecules floating around in your blood!

How does the body accomplish that incredible feat, you ask?

It does so largely by secreting *stress hormones* to *cannibalize your own muscle tissue*, breaking down the proteins in your muscles into amino acids and sending them to the liver where they are converted (via gluconeogenesis) into sugar. This ability is vital to our survival during times when we do not have regular access to food and carbohydrates (like during times of famine or starvation). But when our body is forced to rely chronically on gluconeogenesis for sugar (like with low-carb diets), research indicates that this frequently results in damaging effects on measures of cortisol, testosterone, thyroid hormone (the main hormone that powers our metabolism), as well as, more generally, overall mood and performance.[348 349 350 351 352 353] It is most definitely *not* a state of optimal physiology, as low-carb advocates like to wishfully believe.

Importantly, it turns out that the process of gluconeogenesis is essentially going on *all the time* in our bodies—that is, it is an "always on" process—and it essentially just gets shut off whenever carbs are available. That is, after you consume a carbohydrate-containing meal, the body doesn't have to make sugar from your muscles, so the gluconeogenesis machinery gets to take a break. The rest of the time, the body is essentially *always* producing new sugars to enter the bloodstream. Why is this such an important fact? **Because our bodies are wired to make sure that sugar is *always* available for our cells to run on by always running gluconeogenesis to ensure that there is a steady supply of glucose entering the bloodstream at all times, regardless of what food you are or aren't eating.**

And this is where the logic of the low-carb gurus has become utterly twisted, pseudoscientific, and basically delusional. They have interpreted the body's ability to survive in the absence of dietary carbohydrates as meaning "carbs are not important and your body doesn't need them." But in reality, carbohydrates are so essential to life that **our bodies have been designed by evolution to *still* be able to run on carbohydrates even when we're not eating any!**

---

348 Brinkworth GD, et al. Long-term Effects of a Very Low-Carbohydrate Diet and a Low-Fat Diet on Mood and Cognitive Function. Arch Intern Med. 2009;169(20):1873-1880

349 Spaulding SW, et al. Effect of caloric restriction and dietary composition of serum T3 and reverse T3 in man. J Clin Endocrinol Metab. 1976 Jan;42(1):197-200.

350 Serog P, et al. Effects of slimming and composition of diets on V02 and thyroid hormones in healthy subjects. Am J Clin Nutr. 1982;35(1):24-35.

351 Anderson KE, et al. Diet-hormone interactions: protein/carbohydrate ratio alters reciprocally the plasma levels of testosterone and cortisol and their respective binding globulins in man. Life Sci. 1987 May 4;40(18):1761-8.

352 http://www.ncbi.nlm.nih.gov/pubmed/18951908

353 Lane AR, Duke JW, Hackney AC. Influence of dietary carbohydrate intake on the free testosterone: cortisol ratio responses to short-term intensive exercise training. Eur J Appl Physiol. 2010 Apr;108(6):1125-31.

In other words, carbohydrates are so essential to our health that our bodies have learned to manufacture them in order to protect against periods where we are not consuming them in the diet.

Moreover, there *are* actually numerous negative side effects of chronically consuming too few carbohydrates in the diet! (Many of these are outlined in this series of articles from Paul Jaminet, author of the *Perfect Health Diet,* on Carbohydrate Deficiency: Part I, Part II, Part III, Part IV.) We will also be exploring many of the common side effects of low-carb diets—of which there are many—in the next chapter. But it is simply unquestionable that our bodies do not function optimally with extreme carbohydrate restriction, and that health side effects *do* emerge from chronic and extreme low-carbohydrate diets—even despite our body's ability to manufacture carbohydrates during periods of inadequate dietary carbohydrate intake. **So yes, you can be deficient in carbohydrates, and yes, glucose is essential for the survival of our cells.**

Thus, in order to avoid semantic misunderstanding around the words "essential" and "non-essential," we must consider that there are really two different kinds of "non-essential" compounds:

1) **Compounds that are not essential due to the fact that they are not needed in any way for cells to function normally.** These are substances that may have physiological effects, but are in no way required by the body to stay alive and are not produced by the body in the absence of their inclusion in the diet. (Examples of this might be artificial sweeteners or artificial colors, or MSG, or cocaine.)
2) **Compounds that are *so essential to cellular function* that evolution has wired our biology to be able to function on that substance whether or not it is present in the diet.** (Examples of this are things that may be consumed in the diet, but are so vital that our bodies have developed their own production systems. Things like cholesterol, saturated fats, albumin, numerous amino acids, vitamin D, glutathione, and carbohydrates.)

Carbohydrates fall into the latter category. Yet, low-carb gurus play semantic games with the physiology term "essential" to imply that it's the former. At best, this is ignorance. And at worst, trickery.

In reality, those "non-essential" carbohydrates are about as ***essential*** as a nutrient can possibly get. In the absence of dietary carbohydrates, your body will pump out stress hormones all day long and literally cannibalize itself 24-7 in order to get sugar for fuel. That's how *essential* carbohydrates are to your cellular function.

Keep that in mind the next time some low-carb guru tries to sell you on the nonsense that fats are your body's "preferred" fuel source and that your body doesn't need carbohydrates.

The simple fact is this: **Glucose/sugar is r*equired* by the body, and it will get that sugar one way or another. If you don't eat ample carbohydrates, the body will cannibalize its own muscles in order to manufacture those carbohydrates. You can do it the easy way or the hard way, but one way or another, your body is going to get the carbs it needs.**

Being in a State of "Fat Burning" Does NOT Mean You're Burning off Body Fat!

Low-carb gurus like to promote the idea that by eating their special low-carb, high-fat diet, you can magically coax your body into the elusive state of "fat burning" that will "cause your body fat to vanish right before your very eyes."

Many low-carb gurus love to go into elaborate discussions of the physiology of "fat burning" and talk of things like catecholamines, glucagon, insulin, adrenoreceptors, leptin resistance, ketogenesis, hormone-sensitive lipase, and other fancy words that would make you think they actually understand a thing or two about cellular health. Then they conclude their elaborate "fat burning" monologue by telling you—in an incredible oversimplification—that carbohydrates spike insulin, which blocks you from being in the state of fat burning, and thus it is specifically carbs—as opposed to calories in general—that prevent you from burning off body fat: "When you spike insulin by eating carbs, it keeps all those fats locked away inside your fat cells, and if you hadn't eaten those carbs, your body would be burning through fat like crazy." So, the natural conclusion based on these simple "facts" of physiology is simple: "Get the carbs out of your diet, and you'll get rid of insulin, turn into an unstoppable fat-burning machine, and be lean in no time!"

Unfortunately, it doesn't quite work that way.

Why?

There is a huge mix-up going on today that's causing millions of people to be scammed out of their hard-earned money every single day: confusing the concept of "fat burning" with "body fat burning."

There is a big difference between being in a state of "fat burning" and "body fat burning!"

Most people—including many of the low-carb gurus themselves—fail to grasp the difference between these two things. But there is an absolutely enormous difference between being a "fat burner" and actually burning off *body fat*.

Understanding this critical difference is very important if you want to avoid being scammed out of money by the low-carb gurus selling you "fat-burning" low-carb diets.

Before we get into the details around this physiology, let's go over some basics to help us understand more about what being in a state of "fat burning" really means. What is it that determines whether you are a "carb burner" or "fat burner"?

Whether your body relies primarily on carbs or fats for fuel is really not as complex as some people would have you believe. First of all, let's get some foundational facts straight:

- Carbohydrates and fat are the two major fuel sources of the body.
- The body is pretty much *always* burning carbohydrates and fat to one degree or another. This is true on nearly all normal diets, and it's true virtually regardless of activity level—whether you are sleeping, jogging, watching TV, at work, or lifting weights.
- One factor that influences whether your body burns predominately fat or carbohydrates is activity. Those who are sedentary or doing low-intensity activity can rely on fat as a fuel source. Higher-intensity activity shifts the fuel source away from fat and towards carbohydrates. Carbohydrates are the primary fuel source for high-intensity exercise.
- **The main factor that controls whether your body burns predominantly fat for fuel or carbohydrates for fuel <u>is the amount of fat or carbohydrates you're eating</u>:**
    - Eat lots of carbs and the body gets really good at both storing carbohydrates and burning off those dietary carbs for energy.
    - Eat lots of fat and very few carbs, and the body gets very good at both storing fat and burning off those dietary fats for energy.

So most people get mixed up at this point and say, "Oh, well I want to be a 'fat burner' so I should eat fewer carbs and more fat so my body relies more on fats for fuel—yeah, that will put me in a state of 'fat burning!'"

And it's true! Eating a high-fat, very low-carb diet does indeed promote a state of "fat burning" better than eating a high-carbohydrate does!

The only problem is that this has absolutely *nothing* to do with how much fat you're burning off your body.

Why?

Because the reason your body is burning fat for fuel is simply because *that's the fuel you're eating*!

In other words, "fat burning" does not mean you're burning fat from your body. On a diet with high fat intake and very low carbohydrates (or no carbohydrates), your body will switch to using predominately fats for fuel and you will be a "fat burner," just as the low-carb gurus claim. That is a scientific fact.

What they leave out—and in many cases, don't understand themselves—is that you're ***not burning any more fat from your body***! The fat you're eating simply replaces whatever body fat you burned during the day. When you eat a diet rich in fat, your body doesn't magically burn through all that dietary fat and then decide to burn all your body fat off as well. More fat is being burned off, but more fat is also flowing *into* fat cells.

Just a few months ago, there was a post on Facebook from one prominent low-carb guru who posted a photo of himself at a restaurant eating a meal. He titled the post "how to be a fat-burning machine," and the photo was of him eating a "burger." I put the word "burger" in quotes because there was no bun. This "burger" was composed of a beef patty on bottom and an elk patty on top. In between those two pieces of meat was a special low-carb surprise—a large stick of butter: Seriously. This is a real thing.

Want to know how to be a "fat-burning machine," according to him? We'll give you a hint—it involves eating a diet composed solely of meat and fat and avoiding evil carbohydrate-containing foods like blueberries, oranges, carrots, and yams at all costs. And it's true! He is a "fat-burning" machine! **The only problem is that the fat he's burning isn't his body fat; *it's the stick of butter he's eating every day!***

That stick of butter prevents the burning of body fat in exactly the same way that a bun of equal calories would've done. But who can be bothered with little details like that, right?

It does sound logical and seems to make sense that being a "fat burner" would help you lose fat. Unfortunately, whether your body is relying more on fats or more on carbs for fuel actually says *nothing* about how much fat you're burning off your body.

This is largely a semantic misunderstanding because we use the same term ("fat burning") to describe both the state of using

predominately fat as a fuel source and actually burning off *body fat.* Thus, people get these two very different things very mixed up. People hear "fat burner" and they think "body fat burning."

Simply put, if you're eating 2,000 calories a day of dietary fat on your high-fat, low-carb diet, you have to burn through those 2,000 calories of fat before you ever touch the fat that was in your fat cells before you ate that meal. You know, in *exactly* the same way you would have to burn through 2,000 calories of carbohydrates.

So you might be thinking at this point, "But if I'm not a 'fat burner,' how am I supposed to lose fat off my body?"

Well, the simple answer is this: It is *not* whether your body uses fats or carbs as its dominant fuel source that determines how much fat you lose. It's the total amount of *calories that you consume and burn off each day* that determines how much fat off your body is lost.

This is why, for example, many low-carb gurus are still overweight after years of strict carbohydrate avoidance, and many others don't lose any fat despite years of extreme ketogenic dieting.

You can be the greatest "fat burner" around—someone eating zero carbs, so you are burning almost nothing but fat all day long every day—but so long as you're eating an amount of calories that is at or above the amount of calories you burn each day, the fat you're "burning" is *the dietary fat you're eating, not fat from your body!*

Most people don't realize it, but any time you eat a low-carb diet, by default, that means you have to eat a high-fat diet. Why? Simple—there are only three macronutrients: protein, carbohydrates, and fat. And really only two of those—carbs and fat—are used efficiently by your cells as energy. Your body is burning hundreds or thousands of calories each day—it has to get those calories from somewhere. If you restrict carbohydrates, are you going to have a diet solely composed of protein? No, of course not—you'll realize very quickly that you won't feel or function very well eating like that. You need either carbs or fat to function—these are the two primary fuel sources of your body. If you restrict one, the other has to go up. When carbs go down, you must compensate by eating more fat.

Basically, a low-carb diet is just about switching out carbohydrate calories for fat calories. In other words, if you want to eat a low-carb diet, what's really going to happen is that you're going to eat a low-carb, *high-fat* diet.

Now that you've switched out a large portion of carbohydrate calories for fat calories and made yourself into a "fat burner," you can expect lots of fat loss, right?

Wrong.

As long as calories haven't changed, high-carb, low-fat diets and low-carb, high-fat diets cause—get ready for it—absolutely *no* difference in fat loss. None.

Let us explain it this way. Let's take a hypothetical person—let's call her Sally—and let's say that Sally normally burns 2,000 calories per day. Let's put Sally on four different diets and see what happens in each case: Diet 1 is a 2,000-calorie high-fat, zero-carbohydrate diet. Diet 2 is a 2,000-calorie high-carb, low-fat diet. Diet 3 is a 1,500-calorie high-fat, zero-carbohydrate diet. Diet 4 is a 1,500-calorie high-carb, low-fat diet. Let's take a look and see what happens in each case:

DIET	CARB BURNER OR FAT BURNER	RESULT
Diet 1 – 2,000 calories on a high-fat, zero-carb diet	Fat Burner	No bodyfat lost
Diet 2 – 2,000 calories on a high-carb, low-fat diet	Carb Burner	No bodyfat lost
Diet 3 – 1,500 calories on a high-fat, zero-carb diet	Fat Burner	500 calories worth of bodyfat lost
Diet 4 – 1,500 calories on a high-carb, low-fat diet	Carb Burner	500 calories worth of bodyfat lost

The bottom line is this: eat 1,500 calories while on a high-carb, low-fat diet, and eat 1,500 calories on a high-fat, low-carb diet, and you'll lose the *exact* same amount of body fat, assuming that you're burning 2,000 calories per day.

This fact was driven home recently by nutrition professor, Mark Haub, who did a weight loss experiment where he lost 27 pounds in 10 weeks eating nothing but Twinkies and other processed dessert cakes.[354] He simply put himself in a big caloric deficit, and despite eating pretty much the unhealthiest foods in existence, he lost lots of weight. Clearly, calories, not carbohydrates or insulin, dictate fat loss results.

It is *calories* that determine the amount of fat lost off your body, not whether you are in a chronic state of "fat-burning" dominance or not.

(Note: There is a difference between saying that calories matter, and saying that forcibly restricting calories is a good approach to fat loss. To be clear, yes, calories do matter. However, as discussed extensively in the book *Forever Fat Loss*, forced calorie deprivation does not lead to sustainable fat loss for most people. There is a big difference between deliberate/forced calorie restriction—which research proves has a terrible long-term success rate—and natural, unforced calorie restriction that comes as a result of factors that act to drive down the body fat set point. This will be explained more in the final chapter of this book.)

In addition, it's also important to note that the proportion of carb burning to fat burning doesn't really change much in the context of most normal diets. Apart from extreme types of diets—such as eating a diet with close to zero carbohydrates each day and a huge amount of dietary fat, or a diet of 95% carbohydrates and basically zero fat—there is actually minimal effects on the body as to what fuel sources it's using. The body is still going to use roughly the same proportions of carbs and fat as fuel each day. It is only in extreme diets—eating extremely minimal carbohydrates and eating an almost entirely protein and fat-based diet—that you would even get a significant effect of making you more of a "fat burner."

But again, even if you do enough to get yourself into this elusive state of "fat burning" by eating a diet where 65% or more of your calories are coming from fat, it still doesn't afford any special benefit.

---

354 http://www.cnn.com/2010/HEALTH/11/08/twinkie.diet.professor/

If you're eating 1,500 or 2,000 calories of dietary fat each day, what makes you think that the fat your body is "burning" is anything other than those 1,500-2,000 calories of fat you're eating? Unfortunately for you, that extreme "fat-burning" diet of yours isn't doing anything to actually help you lose body fat. You've just replaced carbohydrate calories with fat calories. **The net amount of fat left in your fat cells at the end of the day is the same either way.**

Contrary to popular belief, burning fat for fuel is not some mystical state of physiology that scientists are still trying to figure out how to induce. Fat burning isn't exactly some mysterious phenomenon that requires magical "fat-burning" supplements and diets or top-secret "fat-burning" diet tricks. Putting your body into chronic "fat-burning" dominance is actually quite easy to do and is very straightforward. We can show you how to be a "fat burner" quite easily. Here is the amazing, secret recipe for becoming a fat-burning machine:

Get rid of the carbohydrates in your diet and replace them with fat calories. Depriving your body of its preferred fuel source (carbs) while giving it lots of fat will force your body to use fat for fuel.

So now you're a "fat burner." So what? What does that actually mean as far as benefits you can expect?

Precisely nothing!

You'll just be burning the fat you're eating—not burning off body fat—but you at least get the benefit of referring to yourself as a "fat-burning machine!"

The simple fact is that for regular people, there is no clear scientific evidence that being a "fat burner" is superior for virtually *anything*. Not health, not vitality, not energy levels, not hormonal health, not metabolic rate, not endurance, certainly not any high-intensity physical activity, and not fat loss.

As we have outlined throughout this book, there is no evidence to suggest that low-carb diets are superior to higher-carb diets of equal calories and protein content. The overwhelming preponderance of scientific evidence indicates that well-designed higher-carbohydrate diets are as effective, or more effective, in every area from health to fat loss. (The only time this changes is in a few specific conditions such as epilepsy, which will be examined in the next chapter.)

So you can make yourself into a "fat burner" by eating a very low-carbohydrate, high-fat diet. Just don't expect to notice any health, performance, or fat loss benefits from doing so.

The bottom line is this: do not confuse "fat burning" with "body fat burning"—they are totally different things. Being a "carb burner" or "fat burner" has no relevance to how much body fat you lose.

SUMMARY

- **Based on an analysis of past and contemporary hunter-gatherers, there is simply no scientific basis whatsoever to suggest that a low-carbohydrate diet was the diet of our Paleolithic ancestors, or that it is the optimal diet for which our genes are designed.** This idea is simply nonsense that has been perpetuated through a combination of fantasy, wishful thinking, and cherry-picking specific populations in support of one's pet theories.
- Ketosis is NOT our default or "preferred" physiological state.
- There is no body of scientific evidence showing that burning fat or ketones for fuel is "preferred" by our cells over carbohydrates. In fact, if there is to be a battle of macronutrient bigotry, the actual physiological evidence clearly shows that carbohydrates would win that title of being the "preferred" fuel source since our cells preferentially use carbohydrates when they are available. This is an undebatable fact.
- The myth that carbohydrates are not "essential" is built on playing semantic games and intentionally misleading people about basic facts of physiology. This is most definitely not a case of "the body can live without dietary carbohydrates, so they must not be all that important." The reality is that carbohydrates are so essential to the health of our cells that our bodies have elaborate physiological mechanisms built into them by evolution that are designed to ensure a constant supply of carbohydrates to the cells even when the body is being starved. Carbohydrates are so essential to our cells that our body will literally begin to cannibalize itself in order to provide sugar to fuel the cells.
- Being in a state of "fat burning" does NOT mean you're burning off body fat!
  - Any low-carb gurus either intentionally or ignorantly conflate the concept of burning fat for fuel with burning fat off your body—deliberately misleading

people into confusing the fat-burning state that takes place as a result of eating a high-fat diet as equating to losing more body fat. These two things have no relationship. The science has conclusively proved that diets high in fats and low in carbohydrates have precisely equal amounts of fat loss as high-carb, low-fat diets when the diets are of equal calories. Being a "fat burner" just means you're burning all the fat you're eating—not that you're in some magical state of physiology where your body decides to burn off all your body fat.

- There is simply no body of scientific evidence to suggest that being a "fat burner" is any sort of "advantaged" metabolic state or that it results in *any* notable health, performance, or fat loss benefits.

Chapter 7: When Low-Carb Diets May be Appropriate

The purpose of this book is to scientifically debunk the myths around carbohydrates that are damaging people's health. It is not to promote any other specific diet, nor is it to say that "low-carb diets are terrible for everyone." Thus, while treatment of certain disease states is not a central focus of this book, we would be remiss if we did not mention the potential therapeutic applications of low-carb ketogenic diets. This is, in our opinion, the only place where we feel the scientific evidence actually warrants the use of low-carb diets. Low-carb ketogenic diets may potentially be useful for treating certain conditions such as epilepsy, neurological diseases such as Parkinson's and Alzheimer's, and, potentially, some forms of cancer. To some extent, this is being generous, and some nutrition experts, **such as Alan Aragon, state the case for low-carb diets even less generously: "[A] ketogenic diet, one that is very low in carbohydrates and therefore higher in fat, is useful for treating some children with epilepsy. That's the only clinical condition that a keto diet makes sense for."**[355] Aragon also notes that "a ketogenic diet is nothing you prescribe universally. Some people can do well because they prefer a fatty diet, but that would represent the minority of the population."[356]

---

355 http://www.askmen.com/sports/foodcourt/high-fat-diets.html

356 http://www.askmen.com/sports/foodcourt/high-fat-diets.html

Research exploring the effects of diet manipulation is ongoing and promising in areas related to epilepsy, neurodegenerative diseases, and some cancers. In some cases, the research shows that ketogenic diets do indeed have specific positive effects. We fully support these efforts and look forward to any findings that can bring relief to those suffering from these conditions—including applications of low-carb ketogenic diets.

One other area of note is that for obese persons who are unable to be physically active (due to complications from obesity/metabolic disease or physical disability), their carbohydrate needs are lower. Some of these people may in fact find that low-carb, high-fat diets are a suitable means of losing weight—at least in the short term. Initial, quick weight loss may help transition them to greater metabolic health and permit increased physical activity. Once able to exercise moderately, a more sustainable balanced diet can be used for further weight loss.

As mentioned in previous chapters, the research is clear that diet adherence rather than macronutrient composition is the crux of lasting fat loss. So it's worth noting that low-carb diets are about as effective for fat loss as other types of diets, and if you are someone who finds it easier to adhere to a high meat or high-fat diet with very low intake of carbohydrate foods, then a low-carb diet may be appropriate in that circumstance as well.

There is also some new research from Jacob Wilson suggesting that ketogenic diets may be effective for improving body composition in resistance-training males.[357] However, the fact that the effect size of this study was so radically different from other studies on ketogenic diets--this one showing improvements far beyond most studies on the topic--gives us pause. The research must be looked at as a whole rather than cherry-picked, and numerous other studies have failed to show such fat loss effects from carbohydrate restriction in general, and even

357 http://www.jissn.com/content/11/S1/P40

in the extreme of ketogenic diets where people derive fewer than 5% of their calories from carbohydrates. [358 359 360 361 362 363 364 365]

Even though low-carb/ketogenic diets may be beneficial in a few very specific circumstances—and that they may eventually prove to be of benefit in certain other conditions—we must point out three fallacies of logic that low-carb gurus often promote.

1) If a ketogenic diet treats a certain condition, then that must mean that eating carbohydrates *caused* the condition.

This is a common error of logic that is often made. Here's an example:

> "A low-carb diet is effective for treating type 2 diabetes. Therefore, eating too many carbohydrates led to this condition in the first place."
>
> "If removing wheat from one's diet causes them to lose fat, then wheat is the cause of fat gain." (A la the book, *Wheat Belly*.)
>
> "If removing grains from the diet or eating a low-carb ketogenic diet helps certain neurological diseases, then carbs must be causing neurological disease." (A la the book, *Grain Brain.)*

Why is this an error of logic?

Well, to stick with the diabetes example, we also have evidence from numerous studies that ultra-*high*-carbohydrate vegan diets can reverse insulin resistance and cure diabetes.

Should we then say it's fat or animal proteins that cause diabetes?

Obviously not. The logic is flawed. Just because something works as a treatment doesn't mean the opposite of that treatment is what caused the disease in the first place.

---

358 http://www.ncbi.nlm.nih.gov/pubmed/15867892

359 http://ajcn.nutrition.org/content/68/6/1157.full.pdf,

360 http://www.ncbi.nlm.nih.gov/pubmed/8363199

361 http://www.ncbi.nlm.nih.gov/pubmed/11374180

362 http://ajcn.nutrition.org/content/63/2/174.abstract

363 http://www.ncbi.nlm.nih.gov/pubmed/2319073)

364 (http://www.ncbi.nlm.nih.gov/pubmed/16403234)

365 (http://www.ncbi.nlm.nih.gov/pubmed/16685046)

If statin drugs work to decrease rates of heart disease, would we then say that the heart disease epidemic is caused by a deficiency in statin drugs in our bodies?

To take this logic to the level of absurdity, if chemotherapy works to treat cancer, is cancer caused by a deficiency in chemotherapy? Should we give out chemotherapy to healthy persons in order to prevent cancer?

The use of ketogenic diets in Alzheimer's, for example, is radically different than the use in relatively healthy people whose goal is fat loss or greater vitality. Ketogenic diets for disease conditions are being investigated as therapeutic interventions akin to the use of drug therapy. Effectiveness in these settings does not translate to recommendations for use in the general population any more than cardiac drugs should be used for those with normally functioning hearts. Beware of the false logic that if a ketogenic diet is effective in treating some forms of epilepsy or Alzheimer's, then the same diet is effective in preventing epilepsy or Alzheimer's or other diseases.

2) If low-carb/ketogenic diets treat a certain condition, then they are the *only and best treatment* for that condition.

As noted above, low-carb interventions can be effective in causing weight loss and improving health status of diabetics—particularly for those diabetics who are among the vast majority of diabetics whose diabetes is associated with overweight/obesity. They can also be helpful in managing blood sugar fluctuations—especially for those with permanent beta cell damage.

When looked at on their own—that is, when examining solely those studies that show fat loss and health benefits from low-carb diets—one can easily draw the conclusion that low-carb diets are the best and only treatment for those people. (And many low-carb gurus do indeed suggest as much.)

Yet, if we examine meta-analyses that compare low-carb diets to higher-carb diets that are matched for calories, all of the sudden, the low-carb diet doesn't offer any profound benefits over calorie-matched diets higher in carbohydrates.[366] The magic of low-carb diets

---

366 http://www.plosone.org/article/info%3Adoi%2F10.1371%2Fjournal.pone.0100652

suddenly disappears when compared to other diets of equal calories, which suggests that the amount of carbohydrates in the diet is not all that critical to the result. Moreover, there is ample research to show that ultra-high-carbohydrate vegan diets are as effective in reducing weight and improving health status in diabetics as low-carb diets, such as the Ma Pi studies. (Note: Vegan advocates often like to use this research to say that vegan diets are the one true treatment for diabetics and the best way to reverse diabetes. Everyone has their chosen ideology that they have allegiance to. And everyone seems to like to cherry-pick the data to support their ideology.)

In fact, nearly all of the benefit that diabetics get from low-carb diets is from weight loss—not any particular macronutrient profile. The simple act of reducing body fat mass dramatically improves insulin resistance and markers of health. Any strategy that effectively reduces body fat will induce profound improvement in diabetics—whether that is a low-carb diet, vegan diet, high-carb low-fat diet, or low reward sugar-rich liquid diet. They will all cause dramatic improvement in diabetics.

Overall calories consumed, food quality, and how much body fat one loses are far stronger determinants of one's results in controlling diabetes (and most other conditions) than the macronutrient ratio of the diet.

In most cases where low-carb diets have benefits, lots of other diets of various macronutrient ratios work just as well or better when they are properly designed and implemented.

Low-carb diets work for fat loss. So do lots of other diets that aren't low-carb.

Low-carb diets work for managing or reversing insulin resistance. So do lots of other diets that aren't low-carb.

Low-carb diets work for improving health markers in overweight persons. So do lots of other diets that aren't low-carb.

3) If very low-carb/ketogenic diets improve the health of certain diseased persons, then that must mean that it is healthy for *everyone* to be operating in ketogenesis.

Sometimes this occurs among regular people who, for example, achieve a lot of fat loss on a very low-carb diet and then immediately rush to assume that it was the unique magic of low-carb diets, and everyone should eat low-carb. Or it might be a clinician who has success treating neurological diseases with ketogenic diets and then assumes that ketogenic is the healthiest diet for everyone.

An example of why this is a giant failure in logic is chemotherapy. Chemotherapy can be an immensely valuable treatment for certain cancers—it can cure cancer in some cases. Should we, therefore, assume that chemotherapy is healthy for everyone? And that regular people without cancer should go on chemotherapy to improve their health and prevent cancer from occurring? Obviously not.

There is a big difference between a state of physiology that works to treat certain disease states and the *optimal* state of healthy physiology in normal non-diseased persons.

Extreme Diets Require Extreme Benefits in Order to be Considered

To warrant extreme diets, there should be a mountain of scientific data showing not just that such a diet produces slight benefits, but *extreme* benefits. This is especially true when those extreme diets go against what we know from research is best for health from long-term epidemiologic data—such as the Blue Zone observational data that examined the lifestyle and diet of the longest-lived populations on Earth.

The great majority of studies of healthy societies show moderate-to low-fat, high-carbohydrate diets of whole foods, combined with numerous positive lifestyle factors.

Research on the benefits of low-carb and ketogenic diets certainly *does not* indicate that such a diet has overwhelming benefits for health, fat loss, energy, or performance for most people. Many studies show either the absence of a beneficial effect or overtly negative effects. (There are several prominent figures in the fitness industry who at one time or another have been vocal advocates of ketogenic eating, who ended up doing crash landings and completely tanking their energy levels and their performance.) Moreover, there isn't even any population on Earth—not even the Inuit—who can be verified to be in ketosis, so we really have very little idea about the long-term effects on health of such a dietary pattern. Even if there were populations who have been eating a very low-carb ketogenic diet for their entire life, there is certainly no body of scientific evidence showing that very low-carb ketogenic diets enhance health or longevity.

Thus, there is an important point that must be made in any discussion of extreme diets like ketogenic diets: **to warrant the use of extreme diets that jettison entire macronutrients, we need research showing not just slight benefits, but incredible benefits from doing so.**

And the research on ketogenic diets to date *does not* show much benefit unless you're an epileptic.

If one wants to go to extremes, at the very least, one should choose extremes that have dramatic benefits and a mountain of scientific evidence to back up their effectiveness—not extremes that may or may not have slight benefits, and a body of literature where most of the studies show little to no benefit.

Taking an extreme dietary approach without strong evidence of benefit is just not very smart.

Do You Want to be a Low-Carb Guinea Pig?

Many low-carb and ketogenic gurus who advocate eating diets of between 60-80% fat imply that this approach is science-based and not only proven to be safe and healthy, but healthier than carbohydrate-based diets.

This just is flat-out not true.

As Alan Aragon notes, "The Blue Zones, which are the world's longest-living populations with the lowest incidence of chronic disease, eat nothing close to an 80% fat diet." [367] Virtually all of them, in fact, eat carbohydrate-based diets or, at the very least, include ample carbohydrates in their diet. According to Aragon, **"There is no remotely strong health benefit of getting most of your calories from fat, and especially from saturated fat."** [368]

Dr. David Katz, head of the Yale Obesity Prevention Research Center, also notes, **"There actually are very low-fat diets in the real world, associated with excellent overall health and longevity. There are no such 'low-carb' diets. People often invoke the Inuit, whose diet is low in carbohydrate and very high in fat — much of it omega-3. But the Inuit are not known for long lives, or especially good health. The Okinawans, on their low-fat native diet, are. The Seventh-Day Adventists, on their low-fat native diet, are."**[369]

The simple fact is that there is no body of research to indicate that long-term high-fat, low-carb eating is associated with superior health or enhanced longevity.

There is no body of randomized controlled trials that has examined the long-term effects of low-carb diets, and the long-term epidemiological research on low-carb diets has certainly not come out in favor of low-carb diets.[370] [371] [372]

---

367 http://www.askmen.com/sports/foodcourt/high-fat-diets-2.html

368 http://www.askmen.com/sports/foodcourt/high-fat-diets-2.html

369 http://www.huffingtonpost.com/david-katz-md/nutrition-advice_b_1874255.html

370 http://www.ncbi.nlm.nih.gov/pubmed/17136037

371 http://www.ncbi.nlm.nih.gov/pubmed/22735105

372 http://www.ncbi.nlm.nih.gov/pubmed/22735105

There is no body of evidence to suggest that low-carb diets result in greater longevity or greater athletic performance, and we already know that low-carb diets are no better than higher-carb diets for fat loss when matched for calories and/or protein.

So if you wish to ignore all of these facts and insist that there are some magical health and fat loss benefits of shunning oranges and potatoes in favor of eating meat and/or fat in their place, that's up to you—but the research certainly does not support the idea that such a practice would be good for you in any way.

If you choose to adopt such a diet, you are essentially acting as a guinea pig in an experiment for which science doesn't yet know the long-term effects. Moreover, you're choosing a dietary pattern that is explicitly at odds with everything we know about the diets of the longest-lived and healthiest populations on Earth.

Having said that, we fully support the use of low-carb diets in any and all areas where they are genuinely proven to be superior in well-controlled studies (such as is the case with epilepsy), and we believe in remaining open to the possibility of their benefit in other conditions. As it stands now, the current scientific literature does not strongly support the use of low-carb/ketogenic diets outside of a few very specific conditions.

SUMMARY

- There is ample scientific evidence to suggest that very low-carb ketogenic diets are an effective treatment for certain conditions such as epilepsy and some neurological diseases.
- Low-carb diets may also be useful for very obese people who are either extremely sedentary or physically disabled and largely inactive.
- Low-carb diets are also useful in the short term (days or weeks) for athletes looking to drop water weight in order to compete in a specific weight class.
- Very low-carb ketogenic diets may eventually prove useful in the treatment of certain types of cancer and potentially other conditions, though this is speculative at this time. We believe in remaining open to any area where the research proves benefits of low-carb ketogenic diets. This book is not to claim that "no one in any conceivable circumstance should ever restrict carbohydrates," but rather to say that the evidence that carbohydrate restriction has any sort of benefits is minimal at best, generally has benefits only in a few very specific circumstances, and for many people not only doesn't benefit them, but actually leads to unwanted side effects (as will be explored in the next chapter).
- There are three major logical fallacies commonly perpetuated by low-carb diet advocates:

1) **The notion that if low-carb diets are helpful in treating a certain condition, it means that carbohydrates caused the condition.**
2) **That if low-carb diets work to treat a condition, they are the only or best treatment.**
3) **Because low-carb diets work to treat a handful of disease states successfully, that means that everyone would be healthier in ketosis.**

All three of these notions are simply false.

- Any diet that is so extreme as to jettison an entire macronutrient should have a similarly extreme amount of evidence to support its effectiveness in order to warrant its use. As of now, the only condition where this is true of low-carb ketogenic diets is in the case of epilepsy and possibly also some neurological diseases. It is most definitely not true of general health or fat loss for the millions of people without neurological disease, where the vast majority of studies find little to no benefit (and frequently negative side effects, which will be discussed more in the next chapter).

- We do not have good data on the long-term safety of low-carb diets. The few populations that do eat a low-carb diet in their natural environment have never been noted for their robust health or longevity relative to numerous known long-lived populations eating high-carbohydrate, lower-fat diets. The epidemiological evidence on the long-term effects of low-carb, high-fat diets certainly does not show that they are superior for health or longevity. Moreover, there are few if any populations on the planet that have existed on ultra-high-fat and extreme-low-carb ketogenic diets chronically. Thus, if you choose to adopt such a diet, you are essentially acting as a guinea pig in an experiment of which we do not yet know the long-term effects.

Chapter 8: The Dangers of Low-Carb Diets

So far in this book, we have shown you that virtually all of the ideas thrown around about why carbohydrates are bad are pseudoscientific myths. And we have shown that in general, well-designed, higher-carbohydrate diets perform just as well or better than low-carb diets in every possible measure—from general health, to insulin sensitivity, to athletic performance, to fat loss. To encapsulate all of that in a sentence, we have made the case that eating a low-carb diet is basically a contrived eating pattern with minimal or no benefits. And we have made the case that virtually all of the claims made by low-carb gurus about the benefits of low-carb diets—that they are better for fat loss, better for diabetics, better for health, and better for performance—are simply false.

To take this one step beyond stating that going low-carb is a generally unfruitful dietary habit, there is data and accumulated observations from thousands of people to suggest that for many people, low-carb diets can actually be extremely counterproductive.

There is a paucity of specific studies looking at the ill effects of low-carb diets—largely because few populations on Earth eat a low-carb diet "in the wild." Thus, we do not have many long-term studies looking specifically at health side effects from long-term carbohydrate restriction. Moreover, many of the existing low-carb diet studies have confounding variables such as increased protein intakes, eating more whole foods (and more nutritious foods) than the study subjects' previous unhealthy diet, and eating lower calories overall—all of which cause weight loss, which tends to improve health status.

Nevertheless, some studies on the long-term effects of low-carb diets have appeared to link them to worse overall health outcomes:

- In a long-term study of Greek adults, researchers concluded that "prolonged consumption of diets low in carbohydrates and high in protein is associated with an increase in total mortality."[373]
- Another study found, "A diet characterized by low carbohydrate and high protein intake was associated with increased total and particularly cardiovascular mortality among women. Vigilance with respect to long-term adherence to such weight control regimes is advisable."[374]
- In a 15-year study conducted on 43,396 Swedish women, researchers concluded, "Low-carbohydrate, high-protein diets used on a regular basis and without consideration of the nature of carbohydrates or the source of proteins are associated with increased risk of cardiovascular disease."[375]

Thus, low-carb, high-protein diets (at least those that have not taken great care to ensure that all animal foods consumed were from grass-fed and pastured sources) have actually been linked to decreased health and longevity.

Crowe et al. notes, "While short-term carbohydrate restriction over a period of a week can result in a significant loss of weight (albeit mostly from water and glycogen stores), of serious concern is what potential exists for the following of this type of eating plan for longer periods of months to years. Complications such as heart arrhythmias, cardiac contractile function impairment, sudden death, osteoporosis, kidney damage, increased cancer risk, impairment of physical activity and lipid abnormalities can all be linked to long-term restriction of carbohydrates in the diet."[376]

Professor of Medicine Joel Kahn, MD, goes so far as to say that **"low-carb diets are associated with an increased risk of heart disease such as heart attack and stroke, with increased overall death rates in general populations, and higher death rates in**

---

373 http://www.ncbi.nlm.nih.gov/pubmed/17136037

374 http://www.ncbi.nlm.nih.gov/pubmed/22735105

375 http://www.ncbi.nlm.nih.gov/pubmed/22735105

376 http://www.ncbi.nlm.nih.gov/pubmed/14672862

survivors of a prior heart attack. In my view, a black box warning should accompany all low-carb diets similar to cigarette labeling."[377]

Yet, it's worth pointing out that many of these correlations of negative health outcomes with low-carb diets are based on epidemiological studies (not randomized controlled studies) and thus they are not without flaw, and as some people such as Yoni Freedhoff and John Briffa have rightfully pointed out, [378] [379] this does not mean that low-carb diets are necessarily causing these effects.

But what these studies do indicate is that if having a lower intake of carbohydrates is a way of enhancing one's health and longevity, we can only conclude that such supposed "benefits" are so small that many studies not only fail to detect these effects, but actually find the opposite trend. If carbohydrate restriction does enhance health, at best, it does so very weakly, and, at worst, it actually worsens health.

Then there is the question over the long-term safety of a high-fat, low-carb diet. Few people have adopted this dietary pattern for such a long time that we have studied the long-term safety of it. For example, the American Diabetes Association (ADA) approves the use of low-carb diets for treatment of individuals with type II diabetes as a legitimately effective way to promote weight loss and improve insulin sensitivity. However, the ADA cautions that this approach should be limited to one year due to the general lack of research supporting the long-term safety of such diets.

While knowledge of the effects of long-term low-carb diets is lacking, some studies have indicated that low-carb diets are likely effective and safe for overweight people. Nielsen et al.'s 44-month study found that low-carb diets are safe at least for that period of time, and another 2- year study found that low-carb diets produced as much weight loss and slightly better cardiovascular health markers than a low-fat diet did.[380] The latest meta-analysis analyzing all the relevant

---

377 http://www.mindbodygreen.com/0-16655/your-diet-doesnt-matter-if-you-dont-consider-these-5-things.html

378 http://www.drbriffa.com/2013/01/26/still-no-evidence-that-the-swedes-are-killing-themselves-with-low-carb-diets/

379 http://211.144.68.84:9998/91keshi/Public/File/38/345-7869/pdf/bmj.e5106.full.pdf

380 http://www.ncbi.nlm.nih.gov/pmc/articles/PMC2949959/

studies done on this subject up through 2014 shows that low-carb diets are about equally effective as other calorie-matched diets: "There is probably little or no difference in weight loss and changes in cardiovascular risk factors up to two years of follow-up when overweight and obese adults, with or without type 2 diabetes, are randomized to low CHO [low-carb] diets and isoenergetic balance [higher-carb diets that are equal in calories]."[381]

The point of this book is not to say that low-carb diets are incredibly dangerous and will give you heart disease and kill you. In general, we believe that a well-designed low-carb diet that focuses on nutritious whole foods is probably relatively safe for most people in the long run—and **a well-designed low-carb diet is still probably far better for health than the Standard American Diet!**

The point is that all of the mythology promoted by low-carb gurus about the benefits of carbohydrate restriction and the supposed "dangers" of carbs is a bunch of nonsense, and that low-carb diets are generally about as good as most other forms of diets when equal calories are consumed.

However, the number of anecdotal reports (which can be found all over the internet) of otherwise normal folks becoming quite ill as a result of adopting low-carb diets is astounding.[382] [383] [384] [385] [386] [387] [388] (And if you're reading this book, you may very well be one of those people!) This is even acknowledged by many low-carb advocates, such as Dr. Cate Shanahan, who ran a contest for people to win free books by telling their stories of how low-carb diets have caused chronic

---

381 http://www.plosone.org/article/info%3Adoi%2F10.1371%2Fjournal.pone.0100652

382 http://www.dailymail.co.uk/femail/article-2611658/How-low-carb-diets-wrecked-health-As-women-reveal-suffered-fertility-problems-hair-fragile-bones-YOU-fancy-trendy-high-protein-diet.html

383 http://chriskresser.com/is-a-low-carb-diet-ruining-your-health

384 http://www.cheeseslave.com/why-i-ditched-low-carb/

385 http://boards.fool.com/low-carb-has-ruined-my-life-danger-20452170.aspx?sort=recommendations

386 http://www.paleoplan.com/2012/11-12/ketosis-experiment-update-i-yield/

387 http://www.marksdailyapple.com/forum/thread18377.html

388 http://paleopepper.com/2012/04/does-the-paleo-diet-smother-female-libido/

fatigue.[389] (Although, such low-carb advocates usually rationalize such symptoms as being due to various "other causes" rather than the obvious cause—the lack of carbohydrates.)

As mentioned in the previous chapter, there are some circumstances when a low-carb diet may be appropriate. But for many of us, chronically restricting carbohydrate intake can have numerous unintended consequences.

Chronically eating low-carb can lead to:

- Decreased thyroid output (i.e., a slower metabolism)[390] [391] [392] [393] [394] [395] [396]
- Increased stress hormone output (especially cortisol)[397] [398] [399]
- Decreased testosterone[400]
- Gut dysbiosis[401]
- Impaired mood and cognitive function[402] [403]
- Poor ability to build muscle and muscle catabolism[404] [405]

---

389 http://www.drcate.com/got-fatigue-from-low-carb-diet-enter-contest-win-books/

390 (http://www.ncbi.nlm.nih.gov/pubmed/3573976

391 http://ajcn.nutrition.org/content/35/1/24.full.pdf,

392 http://perfecthealthdiet.com/2011/08/carbohydrates-and-the-thyroid/

393 http://www.ncbi.nlm.nih.gov/pubmed/20091182)

394 http://www.ncbi.nlm.nih.gov/pubmed/11167929

395 http://www.ncbi.nlm.nih.gov/pubmed/16358395

396 http://www.ncbi.nlm.nih.gov/pubmed/22735432?dopt=AbstractPlus

397 http://jama.jamanetwork.com/article.aspx?articleid=1199154

398 http://www.nature.com/icb/journal/v78/n5/full/icb200076a.html

399 http://www.ncbi.nlm.nih.gov/pubmed/22735432?dopt=AbstractPlus

400 http://www.ncbi.nlm.nih.gov/pubmed/20091182

401 http://chriskresser.com/is-a-low-carb-diet-ruining-your-health

402 http://archinte.jamanetwork.com/article.aspx?articleid=1108558

403 (http://www.ncbi.nlm.nih.gov/pubmed/16685046)

404 http://jap.physiology.org/content/109/2/431.long

405 http://www.ncbi.nlm.nih.gov/pubmed/11167929

- Poor athletic performance in high-intensity activities[406] [407]
- Suppressed immune function[408]
- Fatigue and reduced motivation for physical activity [409] [410] [411] [412]

In simple terms, you're likely to feel fatigued, irritable, cranky, and sluggish, while not performing better or losing more fat than you would on a well-designed diet higher in carbohydrates.

Seeing how widespread some of these symptoms are has even prompted some more progressive Paleo authors to publish articles on the dangers of these diets, which you can see on Chris Kresser's website, and from Paul Jaminet. (And we applaud these authors for their objectivity and integrity in breaking free of the low-carb dogmas in the Paleo community and remaining true to the science.)

We have witnessed hundreds of clients and patients damage their metabolic and hormonal health through low-carb diets. It is becoming increasingly apparent that there is an epidemic of metabolic and hormonal dysfunction emerging in the hordes of people who have been following low-carb diets. This is particularly impactful for women—and especially physically active women—who commonly suffer side effects from their low-carb diets, including:

---

406 http://www.ncbi.nlm.nih.gov/pubmed/9232552

407 http://www.alanaragonblog.com/2013/03/13/2013-nsca-personal-trainers-conference-looking-back-at-my-debate-with-dr-jeff-volek/

408 http://www.nature.com/icb/journal/v78/n5/full/icb200076a.html

409 http://www.ncbi.nlm.nih.gov/pubmed/17904939

410 http://www.drcate.com/got-fatigue-from-low-carb-diet-enter-contest-win-books/

411 (http://www.ncbi.nlm.nih.gov/pubmed/16685046)

412 http://www.ncbi.nlm.nih.gov/pubmed/16358395

- A stopped or irregular menstrual cycle (amenorrhea)[413] [414] [415] [416] [417]
- Decreased fertility[418] [419] [420]
- Hypoglycemic episodes and blood sugar swings[421]
- Depression, anxiety, and irritability[422] [423] [424]
- Poor libido[425] [426] [427]
- Disrupted sleep/insomnia[428] [429]
- Dysfunctional relationship with food and fear about eating either fat or carbohydrate[430] [431]
- Cycles of restriction and binges[432] [433]

---

413 http://suppversity.blogspot.com/2014/07/exercise-associated-menstrual.html,

414 http://www.ncbi.nlm.nih.gov/pubmed/22735432?dopt=AbstractPlus

415 http://www.ncbi.nlm.nih.gov/pubmed/10865930?dopt=AbstractPlus

416 http://robbwolf.com/2013/06/20/female-athlete-triad/

417 http://www.precisionnutrition.com/low-carb-diets

418 http://www.ncbi.nlm.nih.gov/pubmed/22735432?dopt=AbstractPlus

419 http://suppversity.blogspot.com/2014/07/exercise-associated-menstrual.html

420 http://chriskresser.com/is-a-low-carb-diet-ruining-your-health

421 http://www.ketogenic-diet-resource.com/reactive-hypoglycemia.html

422 http://paleohacks.com/low-carb/does-anyone-else-get-depressed-anxious-on-low-carb-16375

423 http://www.psychologytoday.com/articles/200404/low-carb-state-mind

424 http://www.bodybuilding.com/fun/8-low-carb-conundrums.html

425 http://forum.bulletproofexec.com/index.php?/topic/1933-loss-of-libido/

426 http://forum.lowcarber.org/archive/index.php/t-440454.html

427 http://forum.lowcarber.org/archive/index.php/t-330950.html

428 http://paleohacks.com/insomnia/what-could-cause-extreme-insomnia-on-a-low-carb-diet-22448

429 http://www.marksdailyapple.com/forum/thread60777.html

430 http://lowcarbdiets.about.com/od/nutrition/a/How-To-Overcome-Fat-Phobia.htm

431 http://www.shape.com/healthy-eating/diet-tips/cure-carb-phobia-carb-cycling-101

432 http://www.drclydewilson.com/topics/restriction-contributes-binging

433 http://healthyeating.sfgate.com/slipped-up-lowcarb-diet-1200.html

- Chronic fatigue [434] [435] [436] [437]
- Poor thyroid function (and a slow metabolism)[438] [439] [440] [441] [442] [443]

In particular, what is frequently found is a condition called "low T3 syndrome," where a person has chronically low levels of active thyroid hormone (T3). This is significant because thyroid hormone is the major regulator of your metabolic rate. When T3 is low, your metabolism slows down dramatically. When your metabolism slows down, you burn fewer calories at rest and you have to eat less and exercise more to continue weight loss or fat loss. As you eat less and exercise more, your metabolism slows down further. This vicious cycle is why many overweight and obese people end up eating very low-calorie diets and never losing weight.

In this condition, a person may have normal thyroid gland function but still exhibit all the usual symptoms of hypothyroidism like fatigue, weight gain, cold hands and feet, and a body that is extremely resistant to fat loss. The reason why is basically this: In a healthy person with a strong metabolism, inactive thyroid hormone (T4) is converted to active thyroid hormone (T3) in abundance. What happens either in a state of calorie restriction or chronic carbohydrate restriction is that instead of being converted to active thyroid hormone (T3), T4 starts being converted into Reverse T3 (RT3). RT3 blocks T3 from doing its job of powering your metabolism. So as levels of active thyroid hormone (T3) drop and Reverse T3 rise, your metabolism slows down and you can get hypothyroid symptoms. To put this in simple terms, carbohydrate restriction tends to slow down your metabolism.

---

434 http://www.ncbi.nlm.nih.gov/pubmed/17904939

435 http://www.drcate.com/got-fatigue-from-low-carb-diet-enter-contest-win-books/

436 (http://www.ncbi.nlm.nih.gov/pubmed/16685046)

437 http://www.ncbi.nlm.nih.gov/pubmed/16358395

438 http://ajcn.nutrition.org/content/35/1/24.full.pdf,

439 http://perfecthealthdiet.com/2011/08/carbohydrates-and-the-thyroid/

440 http://www.ncbi.nlm.nih.gov/pubmed/20091182)

441 http://www.ncbi.nlm.nih.gov/pubmed/11167929

442 http://www.ncbi.nlm.nih.gov/pubmed/16358395

443 http://www.ncbi.nlm.nih.gov/pubmed/22735432?dopt=AbstractPlus

(Important note: Many physicians do not test for Reverse T3 and thus low T3 or high RT3 are problems that are commonly not picked up by standard blood tests. It is extremely common for people who have this very real hormonal problem—and typical hypothyroid symptoms like fatigue and weight gain—to be told by their doctor "your thyroid is normal.")

I have personally dealt with numerous clients who have wrecked their metabolic function from years of low-carb eating. When they initially come to me, they often say something to the effect of, "I don't understand why I am so overweight and can't lose weight—I eat almost no carbs."

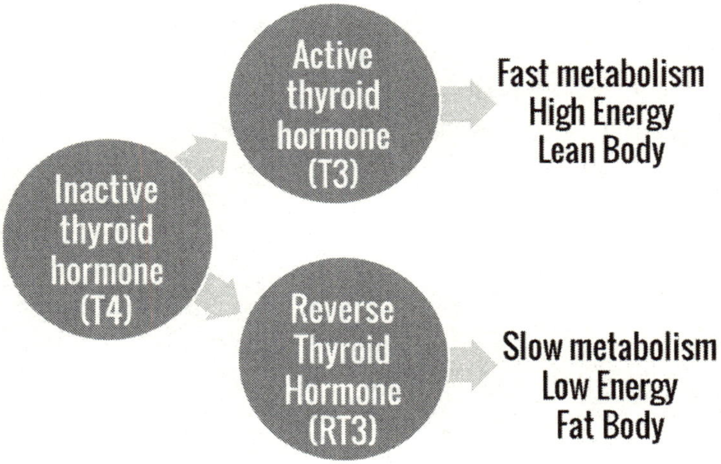

Several studies have confirmed that low-carb diets can dramatically reduce T3 and increase Reverse T3. [444] [445] [446] The consequence is hormonal havoc. Symptoms include fatigue and weight gain, hair loss, menstrual cycle disruption, and other hormonal imbalances linked to

---

444 (http://www.ncbi.nlm.nih.gov/pubmed/3573976

445 http://ajcn.nutrition.org/content/35/1/24.full.pdf,

446 http://www.ncbi.nlm.nih.gov/pubmed/20091182)

thyroid and adrenal function. These hormonal and metabolic issues are becoming epidemic as a result of the popularity of low-carb diets over the last decade.

What makes this phenomenon particularly insidious is that it is occurring mostly in health-conscious people—people who are doing this to themselves because they are actively trying to achieve better health.

To make matters worse, many low-carb dieters have the experience of reaching the dreaded "plateau" where weight loss stops (or perhaps you even start regaining a little) despite severe carbohydrate restriction. Or they start to have the emergence of various side effects like fatigue or insomnia or anxiety. So what do you do then? Well, if you believe that it is specifically carbs making you fat and poisoning your body, the answer is simple: even stricter carbohydrate restriction. Naturally, this is a vicious cycle that actually worsens their symptoms rather than helps them.

Miraculous effects can occur—especially in those struggling with fatigue and hormonal issues on low-carb diets–simply by shifting to higher carbohydrate intakes. The effect is often dramatic in females. Men on strict diets have similar results; however, men seem to be less disciplined in their adherence to a specific diet and thus tend to have suffered less intense effects from carbohydrate restriction. A recent study lends credence to these observations. Researchers demonstrated that in exercise-induced hormonal and cellular dysfunction in rats, the simple addition of more carbohydrate in the diet produced a radical transformation of their hormonal profile, restored healthy menstrual cycles, and rejuvenated the damaged mitochondria of the cells (the cellular energy generators that power the metabolism). [447] [448]

While rat data does not necessarily translate to humans, practical experience has shown that the hormonal dysfunction in low-carb eating in both men and women can be fixed with some simple and tasty medicine: CARBS!

We are not stating that a low-carb diet will always result in these problems, or that a low-carb diet is always going to lead someone into health problems. Many people—particularly overweight people eating a poor diet—stand to have their health and body composition benefit

447 http://suppversity.blogspot.com/2014/07/exercise-associated-menstrual.html

448 http://www.sciencedirect.com/science/article/pii/S2095254614000593)

dramatically from any diet that gets them eating more whole, unprocessed, nutritious foods (which many low-carb Paleo diets effectively do).

And while a foray into lower-carb eating may have initial benefits for the obese individual, these benefits are frequently not sustainable long term. In time, most people find that a whole foods diet that includes ample carbohydrate is an essential requirement for good health, energy, and optimal vitality.

In the cases where people do experience health improvement and/or weight loss after adopting low-carb diets, as we have already shown you in earlier chapters, this is not the result of the carbohydrate restriction itself—it is the result of eating more whole foods, increasing protein intake, and, in general, lowering overall reward/palatability of the diet. (Which are all very good things!)

But for the vast majority of people, the carbohydrate restriction itself is a totally unreliable and misguided approach (based on numerous fallacies and myths exposed in this book) that generally does not result in long-term health and well-being—at least any greater than could be achieved on a higher-carbohydrate diet of equal calories. Worse than that, operating from these myths about carbs—like carbs "make you fat" or "carbs cause diabetes" or "carbs are not essential like fats and protein" or "carbs prevent you from being a 'fat-burning machine'"—is a very predictable way to develop a completely dysfunctional relationship with food while, over time, worsening your metabolism and health.

In general, this is similar to the effects one could expect from a chronic deficiency of other vital macronutrients like protein and fat. If one adopts an approach of chronically and systematically trying to restrict protein or fat intake severely, they are very likely to experience health side effects over time. The same is true for chronic carbohydrate restriction.

The simple fact is that ample amounts of all three macronutrients are necessary for optimal health. Jettisoning any one of these from your diet chronically is likely to result in worse health at least as often as it results in better health.

If you've been eating low-carb for months or years and you find yourself dealing with some of the health problems outlined above, it's time to start reintroducing carbs into your diet!

How to Reintroduce Carbs into Your Diet

Now that we have shown you that all these notions about carbs making you fat or wrecking your health and all the other low-carb nonsense has no basis in reality, you might be tempted to go binge on carbs.

Slow down there! Let's not get ahead of ourselves. If you've been low-carb for months or years, before you jump full force into eating a higher-carb diet, we need to go through some guidelines on how to reintroduce carbs into your diet.

The actual task of increasing carbohydrates in your diet is a simple one: slowly increase your carbohydrate intake over a period of several weeks or months.

However, if you've been low-carb for months or years, reintroducing carbohydrates into your diet can be a little tricky for a couple of reasons:

1) **Low-carb diets impair glucose tolerance.** Many people who have been low-carb for a long time have impaired glucose tolerance. So after they go low-carb, when they eat carbohydrates, they suddenly start to get symptoms (for example, the dreaded "crash"). Many long-time low-carbers experience such a symptom and are immediately re-convinced that low-carb had it right all along, and they really do need to avoid carbohydrates. This is the WRONG conclusion. This is NOT a result of carbohydrates themselves or the inherent metabolic effects of carbohydrates. This is an effect generated precisely because of low-carb diet-induced impaired glucose tolerance.
2) **Carbohydrates impact water storage.** Having higher levels of stored carbohydrates (glycogen) in the body pulls water into the liver and muscle tissues. So in a person who is chronically restricting carbohydrates, we must realize that not only are carbohydrate levels in muscle and liver cells lower, but so too is the water content of those cells. Why is this important? Well, lower water levels in the muscles and liver mean lower overall body weight. When you deplete the muscles and liver of stored carbohydrate, the body loses a significant amount of water and, as a result, overall body weight decreases dramatically. This

effect also happens in the opposite direction—so by refilling the liver and muscle cells with carbohydrate, the body gains several pounds of water weight. To be clear, this is a GOOD thing, not a bad thing. Yet, many low-carbers who eat a meal with ample carbs may notice their body weight go up by a few pounds, and, since they don't understand how glycogen impacts water storage in muscle/liver cells, they immediately have the reaction, "OMG, the carbs made me gain three pounds of fat overnight!" So just as in the first point above, many long-time low-carbers experience such a symptom when they try to reincorporate carbs and are immediately convinced that low-carb had it right all along, and they really do need to avoid carbohydrates.

So first of all, be aware of these factors and DO NOT freak out if you notice any sort of negative reaction to a carbohydrate-heavy meal. It's not the carbs—it's your body having poor glucose tolerance as a result of your years of low-carb eating. And DO NOT freak out if you put on three or four pounds in the first few days or weeks of reincorporating carbohydrates into your diet—we assure you that it's NOT fat, it's just water filling up your liver and muscle cells (which will improve liver and muscle function)! If you are addicted to weighing yourself on the scale and fluctuating by three to five pounds really scares you, we suggest you go back and read the chapter of this book debunking the Carbohydrate Theory of Fat Gain as many times as you need to in order to fully cleanse your brain of the beliefs that carbs are more fattening than fat.

3 Simple Steps to Increase Your Carbohydrate Intake

Keep in mind that this is not an exact science, as we don't have a large body of evidence comparing different ways of incorporating carbohydrates back into the diet after months or years of low-carb eating. But this is the basic template that I have found to work extremely well for my clients to slowly recondition the body to metabolizing carbohydrates normally while avoiding the potential pitfalls of reintegrating carbs into the diet.

Phase 1 - Days 1–10:

Increase carbohydrate intake by 30-50 grams per day and limit use of purified oils/fats.

To add in the carbohydrates, we suggest using berries during this phase (though you can certainly use other fruit, or whole-food starches if you don't enjoy berries). Add in a handful of berries to two of your meals of your normal low-carb, high-fat diet. Try blueberries, blackberries, strawberries, raspberries—anything that you like, and add it in on top of your normal diet. (If you do exercise, a great time to add this extra fruit into your diet is right before and right after your workout.)

In addition, during this phase you want to slightly decrease your intake of refined/purified oils and fats (yes, even the "good fats"), such as cream, butter, coconut oil, olive oil, and any other purified oils you may be using on your low-carb diet. The goal here is not to eat a low-fat diet, but simply to slightly decrease your intake of purified fats/oils while leaving any fatty whole foods (fatty animal foods, avocado, nuts/seeds, etc.) still in the diet just as they would be normally on your low-carb diet. Aim to reduce your intake of refined oils/fats by 1 to 2 tbsp (roughly 15-30 grams or 135-270 calories) per day.

So in this phase, you haven't really made any major changes to your normal low-carb diet—you've simply added some berries (or your preferred carb source) each day, and you're taking in 1 to 2 tbsp less of purified fats, while otherwise eating the same way you normally would on your low-carb diet.

Phase 2 - Days 11–30

During this phase, slightly decrease fat intake in your diet by another 200-300 calories per day, and increase carbohydrates by another 30-60 grams per day. You can decrease your fat intake by choosing leaner cuts of meat, eating some lean fish and seafood in place of fattier meats, and using smaller amounts of fatty foods like butter and nut/seed butters in your food. It is not necessary to dramatically cut your fat intake and eat a low-fat diet. Just decrease your intake of fatty foods a little. If you want to know a more precise amount, aim to decrease your fat intake by roughly 25-35 grams of fat. To give you this in terms of overall calorie ratios, if your normal low-carb diet was 45-65% fat, back it off to 30-50% during this phase.

At the same time that you're doing this, introduce starches and other carbohydrates into the diet to the tune of about another 30-60 grams per day. Root vegetables like carrots, beets, and even potatoes are great choices during this phase. Grains and legumes like rice, quinoa, lentils, and oatmeal work as well if you enjoy them. Dairy—if you tolerate it—like milk and yogurt can also be great sources of carbs in this phase.

Overall, as compared to your previous low-carb diet, during this phase you should now be eating a diet that is 60-110g higher in carbs per day and 10-20% lower in fat.

So if you were eating a 60% fat and 15% carb diet before, you might be eating a 45% fat and 30% carb diet now. If you were eating a 50% fat and 25% carb diet before, you might be eating a 40% fat and 40% carb diet now.

Phase 3 - Days 31 and Beyond

At this point, you should now be eating a balanced diet with more moderate fat and moderate carbohydrate levels. From here, there is no one-size-fits-all solution, so there's plenty of room for experimentation.

If you wish, you can stay right where you are with the macronutrient proportions that you're already at (perhaps something like 30-50% fat, 30-40% carbohydrate, and 20-30% protein).

Or you can experiment with lowering your fat intake by another 10-15% and increasing carb intake by another 50-150g per day (perhaps ending up in a macronutrient ratio of about 20-40% fat, 35-55% carbs, and 20-30% protein. Many people will find this more optimal for energy, vitality, and performance.).

There is room to experiment here and find what YOUR body feels best with. Some may wish to move slightly lower carb, and others higher carb.

One good rule of thumb to guide your experimentation is to first set protein intake, then carbohydrates, then fat.

1) **Set protein:** 0.6-0.8g of protein per pound of body weight; roughly 20-30% of calories is a good estimate for most people.
2) **Set carbs:** Scale up carbohydrates in accordance with your level of physical activity. So if you're very sedentary, you may wish to move more to the lower-carb end of the spectrum of a balanced diet at 30-40% carbohydrate, and if you're extremely active with tons of daily activity and daily intense exercise, you may want to be more in the range of 55-60% carbohydrate. Note that around workout times is an especially wonderful time to take in a large portion of your daily carbohydrates. (As a side note, if you're sedentary, that's NOT good—do something about that and get your body moving! If you absolutely must be sedentary because you are obese and/or in chronic pain or have a disability, you may find a lower-carb diet works better for you. But to the extent that you can move your body, I strongly recommend moving your body more and scaling up your carbohydrate intake in conjunction with that.)
3) **Fat will set itself as a result of #1 and #2 above:** So if you're fairly sedentary and you find you do best with fewer carbs and more fat, you might find that something like 40-45% fat, 30-40% carbohydrate, and 20-30% protein works best for you. If you're very active with lots of daily movement and daily intense exercise, you may wish to go more towards the higher-carb end of the spectrum of balanced diets (20-25% fat, 50-55% carbohydrate, and 20-30% protein).

As I said, there is no one-size-fits-all diet here, and many different approaches within the realm of balanced diets can work wonderfully for the majority of people.

If you're surprised by how simple this plan is, keep in mind that there isn't any need to have some magical or overly complex approach to reintroducing carbs into the diet after eating a low-carb diet with cheat meals and low-carb days and high-carb days or any other such nonsense. The basic rules are:

1) **Eat whole-food sources of carbohydrates** (i.e., choose fruit, starchy vegetables, pure grains, legumes, and dairy, NOT processed junk like cookies, cakes, refined grains, refined sugars, cereal, doughnuts, and soda).
2) **Go VERY SLOW!** Remember those two factors I mentioned at the beginning of this section—the water weight factor and the glucose tolerance impairment factor. So reintroduce carbohydrates VERY SLOWLY! Don't read this book and say, "Oh, so I can eat all the carbs I want" and then immediately increase your carbohydrate intake from 50g to 400g per day. If you've been low-carb for a very long time, make sure to give your body ample time to readjust to metabolizing carbohydrates like normal healthy people should be metabolizing them. Take it SLOW!

If you follow the steps outlined above, you'll do just fine. And if you've been experiencing symptoms on your low-carb diet like fatigue, menstrual irregularities, or other signs of hormonal dysfunction, don't be surprised if you notice that you're feeling better within a month or two of following the steps above.

SUMMARY

- There is very little information on the long-term effects of low-carb diets.
- There are no Blue Zone populations or any other populations on Earth who are consuming a low-carb diet and are known for their exceptional health and longevity.
- The epidemiological evidence on the long-term effects of low-carb diets is generally not in favor of low-carb diets offering health advantages.
- There are several studies and countless anecdotal reports of people suffering various metabolic and hormonal side effects as a result of carbohydrate restriction—everything from increased stress hormone output, to decreased testosterone, to impaired mood and cognitive function, to poor athletic performance in high-intensity activities, to loss of menstrual cycle and fertility, to insomnia, to low thyroid function and slow metabolic rate, to chronic fatigue.

- If you've been on a low-carb diet for months or years and now find yourself dealing with any of the above side effects, reintroducing more whole food carbohydrates into your diet is likely to help you tremendously.
- **When reintroducing carbohydrates into your diet, be aware that carbohydrates influence water weight and that low-carb diets will likely have damaged your glucose tolerance. So take care to reintroduce carbohydrates very slowly, to use whole-food carbohydrates, and to simultaneously reduce intake of fatty foods in proportion to the reintroduction of carbohydrates.**

Chapter 9: The Real Nutritional Factors that Determine Your Fat Loss Destiny

"If you focus on real food, nutrients tend to take care of themselves."[449]

- David Katz, MD, director of Yale's Prevention Research Center

Many of you who are reading this book are no doubt interested in losing fat and maximizing overall health. So we do not want to leave you with our only advice being, "Don't eat a low-carb diet." We urge you to consider a *better* alternative to optimal health and a lean body that will allow you to stop worrying about how many carbs or fat grams you're consuming.

We're not going to offer a one-size-fits-all diet and meal plan, since—as we explain in factor number seven of this chapter—each individual's diet must be personalized and tailored to the individual's lifestyle, personality, and goals in order to be sustainable and successful in the long run. Moreover, our hope is that this book will be something much more than just another "here's the best diet and here's our list of 'good foods' and 'bad foods'" type of diet book. So rather than do what every other diet book in existence does by giving you some one-size-fits-all restrictive diet, our goal here is to offer you the scientific principles of successful and sustainable nutrition for fat loss, as well as guidelines on how to tailor those strategies to your needs as an *individual.* That's the difference between adopting yet another highly restrictive and unsustainable fad diet (and failing), and intelligently

449 http://www.phillymag.com/be-well-philly/2014/03/26/ditch-diet-now/

implementing sustainable and science-based changes in your life (and succeeding). **Our goal here is not to advocate any specific known diet or prescribe any specific macronutrient ratio. Rather, it's to allow you to escape the trap of falling into more unsustainably restrictive diets and yo-yoing in weight by empowering you with the knowledge of the *real dietary factors* that determine your fat loss (and health) destiny. From there, it's up to you to take those principles and strategically apply them in the specific ways that work for you.**

Before we get into those specific nutritional factors, we feel that it's important to remind you once again that fat loss encompasses far more than *just nutrition*, and we strongly encourage you to avoid nutrition myopia (myopically approaching your health and body composition as *solely* a matter of nutrition or solely a matter of "diet and exercise"). Other factors like circadian rhythm and NEAT are just as important to address as nutrition. (If you'd like to learn more about these incredibly important non-diet and non-exercise factors that affect body fatness, we recommend taking the free test HERE to determine which factors are holding back your fat loss efforts, and reading the free accompanying e-book that you're sent out after completing the test.)

For our purposes, since this book is largely about nutrition, we will focus here specifically on the *nutritional* habits that lead to better fat loss results.

With that said, here are the seven critical nutrition factors that are far more important—for both health and fat loss—than the amount of fat or carbs you're eating.

The 7 Nutrition Factors that Are Far More Important for Health and Fat Loss than How Much Fat or Carbs You Eat

1) FOOD REWARD

If you don't immediately know what "food reward" means, make sure you go back and read Chapter 3, where this incredibly important concept is discussed in detail.

Food reward is the single most important nutritional factor to address if your goal is sustainable fat loss. Much more important than your macronutrient ratios, whether you're a "carb burner" or "fat burner," more important than conscious attempts to modify your calorie intake, more important than whether such and such food is toxic, more important than the hormonal effects of any food—simply put, it is more important than *every* other potential nutritional factor you can dream up.

When you eat a diet rich in highly rewarding processed food, your brain's appetite regulation center frequently becomes dysfunctional. The result of this dysfunction is simple: you start eating in order to give yourself neurological pleasure rather than eating because your body requires fuel.

Your eating behaviors become *progressively dissociated from eating according to your body's biological need,* and this means big problems. As a result of eating to give yourself neurological pleasure, you become numb to the signals telling you to stop eating and instead start listening to your brain's cravings for more pleasure, which leads you to overeat and put on fat.

What are the most highly rewarding foods? Generally speaking, modern processed foods are the most "rewarding"—typically in a combination of refined sugars and fats, mixed with artificial flavorings that are professionally engineered to maximize the reward factor in the brain. Sugar by itself is not especially rewarding, though it is moderately so. Fat by itself is not especially rewarding, though it is moderately so. And artificial flavorings aren't especially rewarding by themselves, either. But combine fats and sugars in a refined form (stripped of natural fibers, for example), and lace the combination with a bunch of artificial flavorings that are professionally engineered with the specific intent to maximize food reward, and, well, you have some extraordinarily rewarding food. If a large portion of your diet consists of these foods, you are likely to get dysfunction in the appetite regulation center of your brain and have serious issues with chronic overeating.

An important note: This effect has nothing to do with carbohydrates, grains, sugars, or insulin, as many low-carb gurus like to promulgate. This is about refined industrial food products that are professionally engineered to maximize palatability and reward.

Remember, we told you that it is specifically factors in the *modern* world that are driving obesity. This has been made abundantly clear all over the world—as soon as a traditional tribal society is introduced to processed foods, they see rates of overweight and obesity go from basically nonexistent to skyrocketing all the way up to levels in the United States. As we eat more processed, commercially prepared foods, we consume more overall calories, and as we consume more calories, we get fatter. This trend has been witnessed over and over again throughout the world.[450] [451]

---

450 http://wholehealthsource.blogspot.com/2008/05/ lessons-from-pima-indians.html Guyenet, S. (2008, May 15). Lessons from the Pima Indians. Retrieved from http://wholehealthsource.blogspot.com/2008/05/lessons-from-pima-indians.html.

451 Guyenet, S. (2009, January 19). The Tokelau Island Migrant Study: Diabetes. Retrieved from http://wholehealthsource.blogspot.com/2009/01/tokelau-island-migrant-study-diabetes.html. http://wholehealthsource.blogspot.com/2009/01/tokelau-island-migrant-study-diabetes.html

Food Reward is the Single Biggest Reason for the Obesity Epidemic

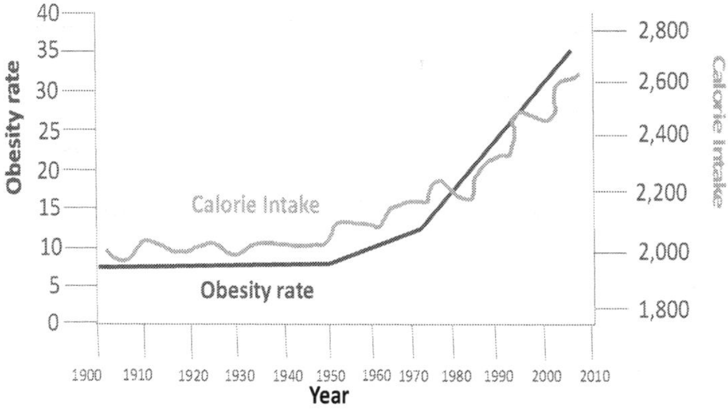

The reason for the modern phenomenon of obesity epidemics in modernized countries is not because people just woke up one day and consciously decided to eat more calories—it's because certain environmental factors (the main nutritional one being increased reward/palatability in the food supply) *drove* up their calorie intake outside of their awareness.

This effect is not driven by the inherent metabolic effects of either fat or carbs/sugar. It can occur either on diets rich in refined sugars or fats, or any combination of them, since they are roughly equally rewarding. As we explored in Chapter 3, obesity epidemics have occurred in conjunction with increases of both sugar and fat, increases of primarily sugar, or increases of fat and decreases in sugar. The key isn't in sugar or fat, it's in overall food reward/palatability of the diet.

While the science around food reward and its physiological effects is complex, the solution here is a relatively simple one:

Eat a diet comprised completely (or almost completely) of whole, unprocessed foods.

This simple step will, to a large degree, eliminate highly rewarding processed food from your diet and allow you to get back into harmony with eating because of biological need, not because you're trying to give yourself pleasure.

This is *the* essential principle of a good fat-loss diet—far more important than conscious attempts to control calorie intake, or macronutrient ratios, or how many grams of carbs or fat you eat each day.

Whole, unprocessed food allows the amount of fullness you feel while eating to be in tune with how many calories you actually ate. In other words, by eating whole foods, you will feel "full" and stop eating sooner than you will with processed foods. This means you will eat enough to be content while eating fewer calories. Thus, no discipline and no willpower to suffer through hunger pangs required.

A recent study showed the power of this simple strategy by looking at leptin resistance in the brain (the primary defect associated with obesity) and how it's affected by diet.

First, they put rodents on a high-fat diet so they became leptin resistant and obese. Once the rodents became obese, they switched them to a 100% unrefined food diet and simply let them eat as much unrefined food as they wanted

Guess what happened?

The obesity and leptin resistance were *reversed*, and the rodents became lean.[452]

This effect is not unique to rodents. In fact, we have numerous human studies that have shown remarkable amounts of fat loss even when people are not forced to eat a low-calorie diet and are allowed to eat however much they want—simply by lowering food reward.

One study found that when they changed the *types* of food participants were eating—even while being allowed to eat however much food they wanted—participants spontaneously decreased their calorie intake from 2,478 to 1,584 calories and lost over five pounds of fat in the first three weeks alone.[453] The reduction in caloric intake was purely voluntary and subconscious, did not involve suffering through hunger and forced deprivation, and occurred while subjects ate to fullness—which is, in our opinion, the key to sustainable fat loss.

Another study found that by changing the types of food eaten, participants *spontaneously and voluntarily* reduced their caloric intake by hundreds of calories per day, such that they burned over 30,000

---

452 http://wholehealthsource.blogspot.com/2014/08/can-hypothalamic-inflammation-and.html

453 http://www.nature.com/ejcn/journal/v62/n5/abs/1602790a.html

calories of their own body fat over the course of the first twelve weeks of eating this way.[454]

Another study found that when eating a specific type of liquid diet, overweight people had remarkable amounts of fat loss (one very obese man lost 200 pounds in 255 days *without hunger)*.[455]

The latest review published in November 2014 identified food reward as one of the "key characteristics of the Western obesogenic food environment due to a highly palatable and varied food supply."[456]

The single greatest predictor of leanness is the extent to which you eat a diet of whole, unrefined, single-ingredient foods that you prepare at home.

This strategy alone—eating only whole, unprocessed foods—has been shown in the research to significantly drive down calorie intake and cause a tremendous amount of fat loss *without* any conscious effort to take in fewer calories.[457] [458] That is the mark of a strategy that is not just starving the body into fat loss but is actually lowering the person's body fat set point, which is *the* critical factor for long-term fat loss success.

Eating whole foods is a simple strategy that you've no doubt heard before, but most people advocate eating this way due to fear mongering over the "toxins" in processed foods. The suggested alternative is to "eat clean," whatever that means—it appears to be defined in radically different ways depending on which health guru you ask.

---

454 http://www.ncbi.nlm.nih.gov/sites/entrez?cmd=Retrieve&db=PubMed&list_uids=17583796&dopt=AbstractPlus

455 http://www.ncbi.nlm.nih.gov/pubmed/5216999

456 http://www.ncbi.nlm.nih.gov/pubmed/25398751

457 Ryberg, M., Sandberg, S., Mellberg, C., Stegle, O., Lindahl, B., Larsson, C., … Olsson, T. (2013). A Palaeolithic-type diet causes strong tissue-specific effects on ectopic fat deposition in obese postmenopausal women. J Int Med. 274 (1), 67–76. doi: 10.1111/joim.12048 http://onlinelibrary.wiley.com/doi/10.1111/joim.12048/abstract

458 Lindeberg, S., Jönsson, T., Granfeldt, Y., Borgstrand, E., Soffman, J., Sjöström, K., & Ahrén, B. (2007). A Palaeolithic diet improves glucose tolerance more than a Mediterranean-like diet in individuals with ischaemic heart disease. Diabetologia. 50(9), 1795-807. http://www.ncbi.nlm.nih.gov/pubmed/17583796

Our recommendation to eat whole foods is not so much about toxins or "unclean" foods or the inherent metabolic effects of processed foods—it has to do with the fact that a diet rich in highly rewarding foods, over time, disrupts our brain's ability to regulate calorie balance in accordance with our biological need and causes us to chronically overconsume calories.

Importantly, food reward is the key factor that can make sense of the simple fact that diets of wildly different macronutrient ratios—everything from Atkin's zero-carb diets to ultra-high-carb vegetarian or fruitarian diets—can produce fat loss. And the fact that when studies compare these diets head to head, they, in fact, typically produce similar amounts of fat loss—regardless of whether they are 80% carbohydrate or 5% carbohydrate.[459] It makes sense of why highly palatable diets of any macronutrient ratio drive fat gain, and why lower palatability diets of any macronutrient ratio will cause spontaneous fat loss.

The *only* way to make sense of this is that the low-carb vs. low-fat macronutrient wars over the last three decades have completely overblown the importance of the carbohydrate-to-fat ratio while simultaneously promoting complete ignorance about the major factor that actually determines whether the food you eat is fattening or not: food reward.

If you're wondering, "How do I know how much food and how many calories I should eat?" consider this from Katz:

> "Do calories matter? Of course they do. (But) the question 'do calories count?' is a distraction. ... The quantity of calories matters—it's a law of physics. But the *quality* of calories—the quality of the foods we choose—is probably the single best way to control the quantity." [460]

And what Katz means by the "quality of calories" is NOT a low-carb diet or a low-fat diet. It is a high nutrient density, low food reward, whole-food diet.

---

459 http://www.theatlantic.com/health/archive/2014/03/science-compared-every-diet-and-the-winner-is-real-food/284595/2/

460 http://live.smashthefat.com/do-calories-count-with-david-katz/

The key principle of an effective diet for sustainable fat loss is *not* the percentage of carbohydrates to fat—it's the food reward/palatability of the diet.

The goal of a good fat-loss diet that will allow you to not just lose fat, but sustain that fat loss, is to cause fat loss while allowing you to eat to fullness.

The fundamental principle to achieving that is eating a relatively low reward/palatability, whole-food diet.

2) FOOD VARIETY

Have you ever been full after eating dinner, having absolutely stuffed yourself, and then suddenly found room for more when offered dessert? Have you ever been to an all-you-can-eat buffet and noticed the "unbuckle-your-pants syndrome" where people can gorge themselves on a huge amount of different foods?

Well, these are both due to something called food-specific fullness or sensory-specific fullness. That simply means that we feel "full," but only for specific foods or flavors. We may feel full on dinner, for example, but not feel full for dessert. We may feel like we've had enough of that savory steak, but we still have plenty of room for sweet and creamy ice cream.

So, as if having highly processed foods that are professionally engineered to maximize neurological reward weren't enough, in the modern world, we also have a high variety of those hyper-rewarding foods. What is the result?

One recent study gives us a clue:

The study is titled "Variety in the Diet Enhances Intake in a Meal and Contributes to the Development of Obesity in the Rat." Dr. Barbara Rolls and colleagues examined the effect of both rewarding foods and food variety on food intake and fat gain in rats. They tested six different diets:

1) Regular rat chow
2) Rat chow plus crackers
3) Rat chow plus cookies
4) Rat chow plus chocolate
5) Rat chow plus crackers, cookies, or chocolate, with each of the palatable foods given in succession (i.e., chow plus crackers, then chow plus cookies, etc.)

6) Rat chow plus crackers, cookies, and chocolate all at the same time

As we might expect, adding a very rewarding food to the diet (crackers, cookies, or chocolate, in this case) increased food intake. Now, here's the kicker: Adding *multiple* rewarding foods together increased food intake significantly beyond just one of the rewarding foods. **So we can see that both variety and food reward contribute to food intake. After seven weeks, the rats eating the high-food-reward and high-food-variety diet gained close to triple the amount of weight of rats eating regular rat chow, and significantly more weight than rats eating just one rewarding food.** [461]

Numerous studies, including human studies, have shown the same result:

> **"Increased variety in the food supply may contribute to the development and maintenance of obesity. Thirty-nine studies examining dietary variety, energy intake, and body composition are reviewed. Animal and human studies show that food consumption increases when there is more variety in a meal or diet and that greater dietary variety is associated with increased body weight and fat."**[462]

People in tribal societies eating their traditional diets eat simple whole-food meals with just a few foods at the most, not three- or four-course meals with lots of different foods to try.

Historically, our ancestors didn't have grocery stores around every corner with an endless variety of foods—they had a very small range of foods that they typically ate day in and day out. The Kitavans eat mostly fruit, coconut, and seafood. The Ewe and Tukisenta eat mostly roots and tubers. The Tarahumara eat mostly corn, potatoes, rice, squash, and beans with small amounts of animal proteins. The Sherpas of the Himalayas have probably 90% of their diet in the form of a meal

461 Rolls, B. J., Van Duijvenvoorde, P. M., & Rowe, E. A. (1983). Variety in the diet enhances intake in a meal and contributes to the development of obesity in the rat. Physiol Behav. 31(1), 21-7.http://www.ncbi.nlm.nih.gov/pubmed/6634975

462 Raynor, H. A., & Epstein, L. H. (2001). Dietary variety, energy regulation, and obesity. Psychol Bull. 127(3), 325-41. http://www.ncbi.nlm.nih.gov/pubmed/11393299

called *daal bat,* which is basically rice and lentils (sometimes with a carrot and potato curry). Over and over again, it's the same exact rice and lentil meal, meal after meal, every day, year after year. **Traditional populations eat *simple* diets and *simple* meals.**

The introduction of different appetizers, entrees, desserts, and endless options of food each day and each meal (especially endless variety of highly processed, rewarding foods) is not congruent with our sensory-specific fullness system and drives us to *eat beyond our body's biological need.* In other words, it's a factor that prevents our body fat set point system from working properly, and over time drives our body fat set point up.

By eating simple meals with just a few whole foods, you have a massively powerful strategy for fat loss. This is one of Guyenet's fundamental strategies for lowering body fat set point.[463] [464] Just as we know that high variety of foods drives up total calorie intake, we also know that lowering food variety (eating simple meals) is an extremely powerful strategy that can cause massive amounts of fat loss that lasts. Again, this is such a simple concept that people have a tendency to overlook it, but if you actually apply it, it's incredibly powerful.

Eating simple meals doesn't mean you have to eat only one food, like a meal of just a couple of potatoes and nothing else, or a steak and nothing else, though such a strategy has been applied by many people successfully, as with the Rice Diet or the Potato Diet. Note that both of these diets are extremely high-carbohydrate diets, and they are notable for their profound fat loss effects. Funnily enough, many low-carb Paleo followers have lost plenty of fat after adopting the Potato Diet![465] This again points out that the fattening effects of food rests minimally in the macronutrient composition of fats versus carbs, and more in overall calories consumed, which is largely determined by the food reward/food variety/palatability of the food one eats. But there is no need to be so extreme, and we're certainly not advising that you

---

463 Guyenet, S. (2012, August 29). Obesity; Old solutions for a new problem. 2011 Ancestral Health Symposium UCLA. Retrieved from https://www.youtube.com/watch?v=srqFz0fO8xk.https://www.youtube.com/watch?v=srqFz0fO8xk

464 Cabanac, M., & Rabe, E. F. (1976). Influence of a monotonous food on body weight regulation in humans. Physiol Behav. 17(4), 675-8. http://www.ncbi.nlm.nih.gov/pubmed/1013218?dopt=Abstract

465 http://www.marksdailyapple.com/forum/thread67137.html

do so. We're talking about limiting your meals to a few foods (perhaps one animal food, plus a fruit and/or vegetable) in each meal and to prepare those foods simply—to not be excessively gourmet and elaborate with fancy sauces and flavorings.

By arranging these whole natural foods in simple meals with just a few components, you are eliminating the possibility of food-specific fullness working against you and causing you to overconsume calories beyond your body's biological need.

This doesn't need to be about depriving yourself of anything that tastes good, or eating nothing but potatoes or meat or cheese. Nor does this mean that you are *never* allowed to indulge in delicious gourmet or processed foods you love—we all need to find the appropriate balance that works for us as individuals, in accordance with our goals and our priorities. You can still have variety in your diet and eat things that taste good. The general principle is to eat whole foods and keep your individual meals simple, and then to deviate from that basic template in accordance with the appropriate balance that works for you based on your priorities and your body composition goals.

It's important to note that eating a whole-food diet should NOT be about restriction.

Given that we already have far too many diet gurus out there trying to give us a list of all the "forbidden foods," our goal here is not to create yet another list of forbidden foods for you to avoid at all costs and structure your diet around. The whole frame of restriction and forbidden foods is a fundamentally flawed approach that sets people up for unhealthy and unnecessarily neurotic relationships with food. Rather than ask, "What should I remove from my diet and avoid at all costs?" a much better approach to nutrition is to ask, "What are the ideal sources of nutrients that support optimal neurological, cellular, and metabolic function?" After you ask that question, then the goal is simply to go about making those foods the focus of your meals—to the extent that is reasonable and sustainable for *you*.

You should absolutely NOT adopt restrictive forms of eating where you feel constantly deprived all the time—this is just a recipe for needless suffering and eventual fat regain.

Please keep in mind that every person has a different level of comfort at various levels of food reward—they have different current lifestyle habits and different levels of desire and willpower for making changes in their lifestyle habits. Some people who are currently eating a diet of mostly processed and pre-packaged food will find the thought of eating a diet of only whole foods utterly ridiculous and undoable. On the other hand, there are countless people already *doing that* without any problem whatsoever—with as much ease and effortlessness as those who eat a processed food diet.

Because of this, there is no one-size-fits-all meal plan that works perfectly for everyone. Depending on your current lifestyle habits and your capacity for making change, you are going to need a different level of food reward in your meal plan.

What you want is to implement the strategies to the point where, first of all, you are actually achieving fat loss, but also simultaneously not feeling like you're suffering (you are not constantly battling hunger pangs and cravings).

In other words, you want to end up in a place where you are eating a very healthy whole-foods diet that is relatively low in food reward, WITHOUT feeling deprived or suffering in order to do so.

You want to be doing this with as much ease and as little effort and struggle as it takes you to maintain your current habits.

(Note: If you want further help with the specifics of how to modify the reward/palatability/variety of your diet for lasting fat loss, Ari Whitten's Forever Fat Loss Formula includes a full cookbook designed by a professional chef along with accompanying meal plans at different levels of food reward—to achieve everything from rapid fat loss to the most easily sustainable body fat maintenance—so you can find the exact set of sustainable fat loss habits that works for *you.*)

To give the basic guidelines, your level of lowering food reward/food variety should parallel:

- **Your desire for fat loss.** If you don't want fat loss and you're totally comfortable with your current body composition, then you don't need to lower the food reward of your diet at all—just carry on eating whatever you like. If you want to lose 90 pounds and keep it off, then you probably need to lower the food reward and food variety of your diet substantially.
- **What you can realistically sustain for the rest of your life.** You should NOT adopt a highly restrictive diet (of any kind) that is unsustainable for you. Cycles of intense and

unsustainable restriction lead to bingeing for many people and, in the long run, lead to getting *fatter, not leaner.* Approach this progressively with small steps that you do NOT feel are depriving or inducing suffering, making sure to lower the food reward/food variety of your diet from the frame of establishing better lifelong habits, rather than looking at it as a quick-fix diet.

- (More on sustainability in factor #7 of this chapter.)

Also worth noting in this context is that the same exact type of dietary habits that are sustainable and effortless for one person to maintain may cause suffering in another person and require constant willpower. So if you want fat loss, you must find the appropriate balance of adopting enough of the habits known to produce fat loss without going too extreme too fast so as to adopt a set of habits that are unsustainable for you, or that causes you to develop eating disorders and cycles of restriction and bingeing. This balance is different for every individual, but we all need to find the appropriate balance of restrictiveness and indulgence that is appropriate for our personalities and our goals.

3) MICRONUTRIENT DEFICIENCIES

The processed-foods-packed Standard American Diet is a micronutrient-deficient diet. It is deficient in countless vitamins and minerals that are essential to your hormonal health and to your cells' ability to produce energy—that is, essential to a healthy metabolism. In addition, it is likely that consuming conventionally farmed animal proteins and conventionally farmed plant foods grown in nutrient-deficient topsoils makes us prone to developing micronutrient deficiencies. Micronutrient deficiency leads to two basic problems:

1) Lowered metabolic rate.

A fascinating study that supports this idea was just published in the journal *Obesity* that showed that, compared to a placebo, a low-dose multivitamin caused obese volunteers to lose 7 lbs. (3.2 kg) of fat mass in six months, mostly from the abdominal region. The supplement also reduced LDL (bad cholesterol) by 27%, increased HDL (good cholesterol) by a whopping 40%, and increased resting energy expenditure.[466] **That's fat loss *without* any change in diet or exercise!** Guyenet had this to say on this study: "This result, once again, kills the simplistic notion that body fat is determined exclusively by voluntary food consumption and exercise behaviors (sometimes called the 'calories in, calories out' idea or 'gluttony and sloth')."[467]

And if you're already overweight, correcting micronutrient deficiencies and supplying the cells with an abundant supply of the vitamins and minerals they need to produce energy will therefore lead to loss of body fat, just as it did in this study. How does it do this? You'll notice in that quote that the multivitamin increased "resting energy expenditure." That means it increased the amount of calories their bodies were burning at rest—at work, while lounging around at the house, and even while they were asleep. In other words, it speeds up your metabolism!

2) Inability to regulate appetite properly.

As Joel Fuhrman, MD's research has shown, micronutrient-richness of the diet has a major impact on appetite regulation, which in turn affects how many calories you eat overall and how fat or lean you get as a result: "A high micronutrient density diet mitigates the unpleasant aspects of the experience of hunger even though it is lower in calories. Hunger is one of the major impediments to successful weight loss. **Our findings suggest that it is not simply the caloric content, but more importantly, the micronutrient density of a diet that influences the experience of hunger.**"[468]

With an ample supply of micronutrients in the diet, the body, first of all, is less likely to overconsume calories and, second of all, has a faster metabolic rate—both of which combine to help prevent fat gain and stimulate fat loss. The micronutrient content of your diet can have profound effects on the calories in, calories out equation.

---

466 Li, Y., Wang, C., Zhu, K., Feng, R. N., & Sun, C. H. (2010). Effects of multivitamin and mineral supplementation on adiposity, energy expenditure and lipid profiles in obese Chinese women. Int J Obes (Lond), 34(6), 1070-7. doi: 10.1038/ijo.2010.14

467 Guyenet, S. (2010). Low micronutrient intake may contribute to obesity. Retrieved from http://wholehealthsource.blogspot.com/2010/06/low-micronutrient-intake-may-contribute.html

468 http://www.biomedcentral.com/content/pdf/1475-2891-9-51.pdf

Let us be very clear: the micronutrient density of your diet is *more* important than the carb vs. fat ratio in your diet.

Does this mean that we are suggesting everyone go out and buy multivitamins to fix all their problems? No. A multivitamin may be beneficial for some, but it's definitely not an ideal solution. What is ideal?

Eat a super-micronutrient-rich whole-foods diet.

No pill can compete with eating a well-balanced, micronutrient-dense whole-food diet. So put your focus on that rather than looking for the answer in pills. The solution is simple: eat a super-micronutrient-rich whole-food diet full of fruits and vegetables, as well as micronutrient-dense animal foods. Eating a whole-food diet could instantly double or triple the micronutrient content of your diet. Specifically, we recommend eating fruits and/or vegetables every single time you eat. Regardless of whatever else you eat in that meal, make sure you get a heavy serving of fruits and/or vegetables.

4) PROTEIN

When people go on a low-carb diet and lose weight, they often think, "Wow, this low-carb thing is amazing. All you have to do is get rid of carbs and you'll get leaner!" What they don't realize is that the same exact thing happens when someone eats a high-carb diet that is equally rich in protein and whole foods.

As we have discussed in the chapter on The Carbohydrate Theory of Fat Gain, the science has shown that when people go on typical low-carb diets, they end up eating significantly fewer calories overall. Why? Simple. As explained, most common low-carb diets are high in protein and in whole foods (thus lower in overall reward/palatability), which are known factors that spontaneously drive overall calorie consumption down.

It isn't actually the carbohydrate restriction that matters—it's the shift to whole foods, the removal of major food groups, and the higher protein consumption driving down overall calorie intake that are the major factors that matter.

This situation where certain dietary changes can cause people to unconsciously lower their calorie intake isn't all bad, though. To be clear—**higher protein intake and higher intake of whole foods are effective strategies to help you reach your fat loss goals.**

If you lost weight from eating a low-carb diet, it wasn't because the carbs you were eating were "making you fat"; it was because you decreased your calories (as a result of lowering overall food reward of your diet) and likely increased your protein intake.

Use this knowledge to your advantage!

Higher protein intake is an extremely powerful strategy for achieving lasting fat loss—due largely to helping to preserve muscle mass during a caloric deficit, increasing satiety, lowering food reward of the diet, and driving overall calorie consumption down.

We recommend putting a focus on <u>eating 0.6-0.8g of protein per pound of body weight per day.</u> This should be your daily goal for fat loss.

It is worth pointing out here that the quality of the protein matters, and there is some research showing that very high intakes of animal meats—at least from conventionally raised (non-grass-fed/pastured) animals—may not be very healthy. So it is likely wise to get your protein from naturally raised and healthy animals. If that's not possible for you, there are many quality dairy, egg white, and vegan protein powders (such as brown rice protein, hemp protein, pea protein, and potato protein) that are available as relatively cheap sources of quality protein.

It is important to note that high protein intake is NOT an *essential* requirement for sustainable fat loss. There are, in fact, many examples of people on lower protein diets (such as vegans) who are extremely lean. This is largely because they have most of the other six factors mentioned here in place.

The research shows us that it is possible to be lean and healthy on a huge range of different macronutrient profiles, from diets that have large amounts of animal foods (high in protein, moderate to high in fat, and moderate to low in carbohydrates) to near-complete vegan diets (which are usually high in carbohydrates and very low in fat and protein)—as long as those diets are whole-food diets that are low reward. So optimizing protein intake is not an essential principle here in the way many of the other principles here are, but it can be extremely helpful nonetheless.

5) EAT LOTS OF PLANTS!

As Michael Pollan famously advised, "Eat food. Not too much. Mostly plants."

Focus on taking the majority of the volume of your diet in the form of plant foods—particularly, fruits and vegetables. The evidence is overwhelming that, second to eating a minimally processed diet of mostly whole foods, this is perhaps the most essential requirement for health.

David Katz, MD, in reviewing the literature on the health effects of various kinds of diets, drew this conclusion:

> **"Yes, I argue that [we should be eating] 'mostly plants,' because the evidence argues that way—not because I own stock in Brussels sprouts. A Paleo style diet that derives 50% of its calories from game is still 'mostly plants' by volume, and a legitimate variation on the theme for those inclined to go that way. But the popular mantra of more 'meat, butter, and cheese' is off the theme altogether. I don't say that because I win a prize every time someone declines pastrami. I say that because it's what the weight of evidence indicates."**[469]

The Lyon study is particularly important to acknowledge in the context of a book examining low-carb, high-fat diets, as it is a landmark study that sets the standard for nutrition research. This randomized, controlled trial diet compared a whole food, Northern European diet (rich in meat, butter, and cheese) against a Mediterranean diet, which is comparatively lower in fat and higher in carbohydrate-rich plant foods. Both diets in this case were whole-food diets. On the Mediterranean diet, they replaced most red meat with fish or poultry, as well as cut out butter and cream from the diet, replacing them with a spread similar to olive oil. Study subjects were specifically instructed to eat more vegetables with at least one serving of fruit every day. **The result of this study showed profound and remarkable benefits in favor of the plant-based Mediterranean diet over the meat-, butter-, and cheese-rich diet. After a little less than four years on**

---

469 http://www.huffingtonpost.com/david-katz-md/study-saturated-fat-as-ba_b_5507184.html

the Mediterranean-style diet, participants cut their incidence of heart attacks by up to 70 percent.[470] [471]

If you're coming from a low-carb diet that is restrictive in carbohydrate foods and instead emphasizes fatty foods, the simplest way to think about what to do is to decrease your intake of very fatty foods (i.e., choose fewer fatty animal foods and less oil/purified fat, etc.) while simultaneously *replacing* those fatty foods with fruits and vegetables.

Focus on making fruits and/or vegetables the foundation of every single meal you eat, and, in general, make plant foods the bulk of your diet.

Katz' comprehensive review of the diet studies—which is one of the single most complete pieces of nutrition research ever conducted—clearly showed the benefits of diets rich in plant foods. After rigorous analysis of hundreds of the most relevant nutrition studies ever conducted, the authors concluded: "The case that we should eat true food, mostly plants, is all but incontrovertible."[472]

6) METABOLIC HEALTH

One more critical factor to concern yourself with is the health of your metabolism. The metabolism is affected by numerous different hormones, from adrenaline to progesterone to estrogen to testosterone to cortisol to insulin to leptin. But the major player in your metabolic rate is thyroid hormone. In turn, your metabolic rate dictates almost *everything* about how well your body functions. With low thyroid and low metabolic rate, you're likely to experience fatigue, to perform poorly both mentally and physically, to have a low libido, to feel irritable/anxious/depressed/moody much of the time, to be prone to putting on fat easily, and, in general, you will lack energy and vitality.

(Note: The science around this topic would fill an entire book in itself and is far too vast to summarize in this section. Ari Whitten has actually written an entire 350-page book--and developed a series of video lectures based on that book--on this topic in his Metabolism Supercharge program. Here we will not copy and paste those 350

---

470 http://circ.ahajournals.org/content/103/13/1823.full

471 http://www.huffingtonpost.com/david-katz-md/bittman-butter_b_5042270.html

472 http://www.realfoods.co.uk/article/the-real-food-diet

pages, but rather we will give you a brief summary of many of the common factors that can impair metabolic health as well as some basic guidance on how to fix them.)

Numerous factors—both nutritional and non-nutritional—affect metabolic and hormonal health, such as circadian rhythm; fatty acid profile of the diet; amino acid profile of the diet; movement habits/sitting; specific wavelengths of light; vitamins A, B, D, E, and K; psychological stress; minerals like copper, zinc, sodium, and magnesium; and blood levels of sex hormones like progesterone, estrogen, and testosterone, among other factors. There are dozens of nutrition and lifestyle factors that can impair the production and conversion of thyroid hormone in our bodies and create poor metabolic/hormonal health. To give you an idea of how complex this area is, here are some of the factors that influence your thyroid and metabolic health:

Low-calorie diets - Chronic calorie restriction is perhaps the surest way to decrease thyroid hormone production, conversion, and utilization at the cellular level. It is just not possible to have a fast metabolism without adequate calories present in the diet. Take in ample calories. You want to regulate energy balance at a HIGH level of calories in, calories out (FLUX)—not a low level. The more you train your brain and metabolism to regulate flux at high levels of flux (i.e. more calories in, and more calories out), the better your metabolic health tends to be.

Low-carb eating - Carbohydrate restriction is known to impair thyroid hormone production. As discussed in the section on how carb restriction can damage your health, chronically restricting carbohydrates will lead to increased levels of Reverse T3 thyroid hormone, which will slow the metabolism. You need ample carbs in the diet to prevent this.

Disrupted circadian rhythm - Much recent evidence suggests that hypothyroidism is fundamentally a circadian rhythm disorder and that nearly all people who produce less thyroid hormone have disrupted circadian rhythm.

Micronutrient deficiencies - Certain micronutrient deficiencies like B-vitamins, vitamin A, vitamin E, and vitamins D and K, as well as mineral deficiencies like magnesium, selenium, and zinc can have an absolutely enormous impact on thyroid levels.

Low-protein diet - Adequate protein is needed for thyroid gland health, and it is not uncommon for vegetarians and vegans to develop hypothyroidism (though excessively high meat consumption may also not be ideal for thyroid health).

Sitting (i.e., movement deficiency) - Yes, sitting itself is a major factor that harms metabolic and hormonal health. The increased blood fats and blood sugar that happen during prolonged sitting and movement deficiency are toxic to the cells (including the thyroid gland) and can impair thyroid hormone production.

High omega-6 fat consumption - High consumption of omega-6 polyunsaturated fats is likely to impair thyroid hormone production.

Goitrogens - Environmental compounds like fluoride, chlorine, and xenoestrogens from pesticides (all found in the water supply), as well as some foods people commonly think are healthy like raw cruciferous vegetables (broccoli, cauliflower, kale, and cabbage) can all impair thyroid hormone production.

Excessive water consumption - Following the typical health advice to consume huge amounts of water each day beyond what the body craves can actually be problematic for many people as it dilutes body fluids and puts undue stress on the kidneys to get rid of the excess water while holding on to vital minerals. Doing this day in and day out results in increased aldosterone levels, which can create excess stress hormones in the body that suppress thyroid hormone production.

Autoimmunity - In autoimmune conditions, the thyroid gland can be progressively attacked and destroyed by the immune system. As the gland itself is being eaten away, thyroid hormone production decreases in parallel.

Overexercising (especially with cardio) - Overexercising can put a great deal of stress on the body, in addition to causing nervous system burnout and excessive inflammation. The science has now shown that endurance exercise (aka "cardio") produces hypercortisolinemia (that is, excess cortisol, which is a stress hormone). Over time, this can cause all sorts of deleterious effects in the body like decreasing fertility (which is why so many female endurance athletes lose their periods and become infertile) and decreased thyroid hormone production.

Light exposure deficiency - Believe it or not, regular exposure of your body (including directly on the thyroid gland itself) to the sun is extremely important for normal thyroid function. Specifically, near-infrared and red light are the frequencies of light that stimulate the thyroid gland to produce thyroid hormone. And we now have studies showing that red light/near-infrared light therapy directly on the thyroid gland is one of the few treatments that has ever been shown to slow (and potentially even reverse) some cases of poor thyroid health.

History of yo-yo dieting - Whenever you do a low-calorie diet, your body adapts to that diet by decreasing thyroid hormone production and slowing down the metabolism. Attempting low-calorie diets multiple times over the years can result in *long-lasting* (i.e., near-permanent) decreases in metabolic rate, so your metabolism not only slows down during the diet, but it *stays* slow.

High cortisol - This has to do with everything from lack of sleep/disrupted circadian rhythm, to stress, to lack of sunlight, to excessive sitting and movement deficiency, to excessive cardio, to lack of recharge time.

Gut inflammation and dysbiosis - This not only contributes to endotoxin entering the blood and decreasing T4 to T3 conversion in the liver, but also decreases T4 to T3 conversion in the other major area where T4/T3 conversion happens—in the gut itself.

Fatty acid profile imbalance - This has to do with seed oils and omega-6 fat consumption, as well as deficiency in other important fatty acids.

An overburdened, glycogen-deficient liver - The liver is the major place where T4 is converted to T3. An overburdened liver that is being forced to deal with toxins (such as alcohol or other drugs and other toxins) does not have ample glycogen stores and micronutrient availability and will be extremely inefficient in converting T4 to T3.

Estrogen dominance and low progesterone - This is a major factor that prevents the binding of thyroid hormones to the cells where they can actually work their metabolism-boosting magic. Estrogen—including from birth control pills—increases thyroid-binding globulin in the blood, which lowers the amount of free thyroid hormone available to enter cells.

Insulin resistance (i.e., excess body fat) - This has to do with chronic calorie overconsumption, sitting/movement deficiency, and micronutrient and phytonutrient deficiency.

Poor meal timing - Regularly going without food for prolonged periods (or without taking in meals balanced with protein, carbs, and fats) can increase stress in the body and prevent efficient conversion of T4 to T3. This also relates to circadian rhythm.

Inflammation - Chronic inflammation is another huge factor that impairs T4 to T3 conversion, and it also impairs the ability of T3 to actually enter your cells—that is, it makes your cells resistant to thyroid hormone.

To get you started in the right direction, here are some principles to follow:

- √ If you are chronically trying to restrict calories because you're afraid that too many calories will make you fat, perhaps it's time to stop starving your body of the calories it needs for your metabolism to run properly (and, by the way, if you do things right to stimulate your metabolism, you should be getting *leaner* while eating more calories).
- √ If you are chronically restricting your calorie intake, perhaps it's time to take steps to raise your daily caloric flux. Take in ample calories and focus on increasing your N.E.A.T. (non-exercise activity thermogenesis). You want to regulate energy balance at a *high* level of calories in, calories out (FLUX)—not a low level.
- √ If disrupted circadian rhythm and poor sleep quality are a factor, take steps to get that corrected.
- √ If you've been restricting carbohydrate intake for a long time, it's probably time to start increasing your carbohydrate intake so your liver can do its job of converting T4 to T3 effectively.

- √ If you've been on a processed food diet or you don't regularly consume foods rich in vitamins A, E, K, and the B-vitamins (which are needed for production and conversion of thyroid hormone), then you need to start seeking those foods out.
- √ If you're chronically stressed, integrate de-stressing rituals into your life.
- √ If you have chronic inflammation, eat more fruits and vegetables that are rich in anti-inflammatory phytonutrients.
- √ If you are sitting for most of the day, take steps to be more active.
- √ If you are an exercise addict and you are fatigued all the time, it's time to shift towards gentler, more rejuvenative forms of exercise—at least for a period of time.
- √ If you're eating lots of raw cruciferous veggies like kale and broccoli on a regular basis, perhaps it's time to start cooking them.
- √ If you're taking in lots of vegetable oils in your diet, time to back off the omega-6 fat consumption.
- √ If your light exposure patterns are off because you spend most of the day indoors and the evening in front of your television, phone, or computer, take steps to correct that. More light during the daylight hours, and less late at night.

7) SUSTAINABILITY

As we have already seen throughout this book, every diet works for fat loss. And they all work about equally well. As this recent meta-analysis that compared everything out there from Atkins to The Zone diets found:

"Significant weight loss was observed with any low-carbohydrate or low-fat diet. Weight loss differences between individual named diets were small. This supports the practice of recommending any diet that a patient will adhere to in order to lose weight."[473]

In general, we already know that diets that vary wildly in macronutrient content can all work effectively for fat loss. And we know that they all work with about the same level of effectiveness.

473 http://jama.jamanetwork.com/article.aspx?articleid=1900510

We know that the crux here is long-term dietary compliance and sustainability—not what the macronutrient content of the diet is.

As researcher George Bray states very plainly and directly, **"Weight loss is related to adherence to the diet, not to its macronutrient composition."**[474]

Indeed, many people in the fitness and nutrition industry look at the simple fact that all diets of dramatically varying macronutrient content seem to work equally as well as one another and conclude: "It doesn't matter what type of diet you choose—what matters is that you stick with it."

And to a large extent, we agree with this sentiment. But the problem is that that's as far as many people go! They fail to consider that weight loss is obviously *not* as simple as "all diets work as long as you eat fewer calories, and therefore, all that matters is that you stick to eating fewer calories."

How do we know fat loss isn't that simple?

Well, although every approach can be said to "work," they also all seem to *not work!*

That is, most diets don't work very well for most people: upwards of 95% of people fail to achieve lasting fat loss.

This is a documented fact. Nearly all people who adopt any sort of weight loss diet end up in failure. They may adopt a new diet or exercise program and lose lots of weight initially, but within one to two years, most people have regained everything they lost and more. Even in the case of *professionally* designed weight loss and weight loss maintenance programs where study participants receive ongoing training, accountability support, and guidance from diet professionals, success rates for lasting weight loss are still abysmal in most cases.[475] Most people *still* regain all the fat they initially lost.

Thus weight loss in general seems to be a rather peculiar problem. On the one hand, the problem of weight loss appears to be an exceedingly simple problem with an unbelievably obvious solution: fat gain is caused by consuming more calories

---

474 http://www.proteinpower.com/drmike/wp-content/uploads/2008/07/bray-review-of-gcbc.pdf

475 http://www.thelancet.com/journals/landia/article/PIIS2213-8587%2814%2970200-1/abstract

than one expends, and thus fat loss is as simple as reversing this situation—expending more calories than one consumes.

Yet there seems to be a fundamental disconnect between this simple way of conceptualizing weight loss and the *lived reality* of those who attempt to lose weight in this way. Renowned obesity scientist Rudolph Leibel, MD, explains this disconnect very succinctly:

> "In fact, when you look at the numbers—and they're hard to get, because for a number of reasons, many of the commercial enterprises don't necessarily want to publicize this—**the recidivism rate to obesity following what would be considered a successful weight reduction is probably over 95 percent.** That can be interpreted a number of ways, but in the context of this biological picture of the process, what it tells you is that it is not so easy to perturb individuals from [a stable weight level] by the expedient of dietary management. **One of the things that is not well recognized is the fact that weight loss itself—that is, the actual ability to reduce body weight—is not a particularly difficult problem. If you put human beings on an 800-calorie or 1000-calorie diet, they lose weight. … But what does characterize the vast majority of humans is that they are very resistant to the maintenance of body weight below whatever 'normal' for them is."**[476]

So why is weight loss so difficult to achieve? If it's so simple, then why do over 95% of fail to achieve it?

One factor here is that most people adopt approaches that are inherently unsustainable due to the radical nature of the approach, or that the approach is actually sold as a short-term quick-fix "do-this-for-30-days" type of weight loss program that the individual has no intention of sustaining for life. Examples of this include very low-calorie diets where you feel like you're starving half the time (as is common in many physician-run weight-loss clinics), juice fasts, cutting out major food groups, cutting carbs (or some other nutrient) to the point where you can't eat outside your home and end up having no social life, and all the "lose a pound a day for 15 days" type of magic pill diets out there. Many of these programs do indeed work to cause rapid fat loss and 20, 30, or 50 pounds will be lost in a short period of

---

476 http://www.scientificamerican.com/article/interview-with-rudolph-l/

time, but the problem is that when we check on these people a year or two later, virtually all of them are as fat as when they first began the diet (or fatter).

Many diets fail because their approach limits many of the most commonly consumed food groups too extremely. It's well established, for example, that vegans and vegetarians often have a terribly difficult time actually sticking to their non-meat eating ways, and at one time or another, most of them end up reverting back to eating at least some animal foods from time to time. Low-carb ketogenic diets that ask people to not only sharply limit carbohydrate intake, but also their protein intake (in order to stay in ketosis), also suffer from absolutely horrible compliance rates. **If the goal is *long-term, lasting, sustainable* improvements in health or fat loss, it's critically important to recognize that the more extreme the diet (the more it is heavily restrictive of one food group or another), the poorer compliance tends to be.**

Thus the notion of everyone eating diets of essentially nothing but fat and protein with only a tiny amount of carbohydrate as a widespread initiative to combat obesity is laughable, since any dietary pattern so extreme as to jettison an entire macronutrient (and simultaneously limit another one) is simply unsustainable for the majority of people.

Even in the major area where we do have good evidence of the effectiveness of very low-carb ketogenic diets—with seizures—many people fail to sustain a ketogenic diet. Research has verified the low compliance rates on ketogenic diets, even when prescribed for severe health problems:

- "For this reason the ketogenic diet represents an interesting option but unfortunately suffers from a low compliance."[477]
- "The ketogenic diet, a treatment for intractable epilepsy, is rarely initiated because it requires strict compliance with a diet that is perceived to be unpalatable."[478]
- "Studies investigating the effectiveness of ketogenic diets are all observational based and focus on the patients that were compliant with the diet; however, most of these studies have

477 http://www.nutritionj.com/content/10/1/112

478 http://www.ncbi.nlm.nih.gov/pubmed/7592151

large dropout rates. In the above meta-analysis, about half of the patients dropped out. Families primarily discontinued the diet due to the lack of improvement in seizure control."[479]

- WebMD explains it this way: "Some parents of children with epilepsy are skeptical of the ketogenic diet when they first hear about it. A diet that can control epilepsy and stop seizures without any medication? It almost sounds like a scam. But the ketogenic diet is real and legitimate. It works very well in many people. The catch is that it's extremely demanding and difficult to follow. In fact, it is so difficult to follow that most doctors recommend it only for people who haven't been able to control their seizures with medicine."[480]

Because we know that sustainability—rather than some magical macronutrient ratio—is the crux of lasting fat loss, any dietary pattern that is found to be so unpleasant that it suffers very low compliance can be immediately ruled out as a real option to fix the obesity epidemic. In the words of obesity scientist Yoni Freedhoff, MD, **"Ultimately the issue I have got with this style of diet—the issue with all low-carb diets—is not that they can't work or help, but for the majority of people who go on them, it's not sustainable."**[481]

Thus, even if ketogenic diets had unanimous support from the scientific literature showing that being in ketosis offered incredible fat loss benefits over every other kind of diet even at equal calorie intakes—and to be clear, they certainly do *not* enjoy that distinction—they would still be irrelevant to the discussion of what to do about the obesity epidemic since we already know that the most effective diets for long-term fat loss are those that people can stick to. In Freedhoff's words, **"Ultimately the best diet for you is the one you actually enjoy enough to keep living with, as merely tolerable diets won't last."**[482]

---

479 http://www.hindawi.com/journals/isrn/2012/263139/

480 http://www.webmd.com/epilepsy/the-ketogenic-diet

481 http://www.vox.com/2014/12/19/7416939/bulletproof-coffee

482 http://www.weightymatters.ca/2014/09/what-i-learned-by-actually-reading-that.html

Any sort of extreme restriction—of calories, or carbs, or any other food group—is likely to be unsustainable for the vast majority of people. **And in many cases, such periods of extreme restriction will actually be counterproductive.**

We have the research that has already shown us that periods of forced deprivation and restriction—whether that is in the form of calorie restriction, food group restriction, or macronutrient restriction—can create bingeing behaviors afterwards and likely promote *increased* body fat in the long run.

For example, one study found that **"weight-loss attempts may be associated with subsequent major weight gain, even when several potential confounders are controlled for."**[483]

So if you want sustainable and lasting fat loss, the first rule is: don't do the extreme forced-restriction diets in the first place!

Another reason why so many fail is that we simply aren't wired very well to consciously control our calorie intake—for millions of years, humans and animals haven't even known what a calorie is, let alone had to consciously monitor their food intake in order to remain effortlessly lean. So it is totally unnatural for our species to be constantly neurotic about counting the calories in each bite of food we eat in order to make sure we don't exceed some predetermined number.

Another reason is that large habit changes of any kind are simply difficult to establish. We are creatures of habit that routinely fall back into old habits.

But perhaps the biggest reason is that when we try to lose weight, our bodies *fight back!* On the surface, fat loss appears to be a very simple thing to do—just eat fewer calories and work out a little more. The problem is that when we try to do this, our bodies fight back with **compensatory changes like hunger pangs, fatigue, and lowered energy expenditure, which act over time to slowly pile the fat back on.**

In fact, our bodies have evolved a system—known to obesity scientists as the body fat set point system—whose primary job it is to do precisely that: to fight against the loss of body fat.

Basically, in much the same way that our body regulates things like blood oxygen levels, body temperature, sleep/wake cycles, and blood

---

483 http://ajcn.nutrition.org/content/70/6/965.long

sugar, our bodies also regulate our level of body fat. When we deviate from our normal level of fat mass, the body fat set point system switches on mechanisms to "defend" the normal level of fat mass. It does this first through simple hunger, and then if you don't eat adequately, the body will engage all sorts of mechanisms to decrease energy expenditure (metabolism slowdown, decreased NEAT, and lethargy).

Why did this system evolve?

Simple. Having a system built into your biology that allows you decrease your energy expenditure during times of low calorie intake is immensely valuable for surviving inevitable periods of famine or food shortage. In other words, it's not a mistake that we have evolved this system—it is what allowed our ancestors to survive.

The basic way that your body tries to keep a stable bodyweight:

	HUNGER	METABOLISM	RESULT
PERIOD OF OVEREATING	↓	↑	Bodyweight stays stable
PERIOD OF UNDEREATING	↑	↓	Bodyweight stays stable

The "burn more calories than you take in" approach to fat loss fails to achieve lasting fat loss because when you eat fewer calories, the body decreases calorie burning in an effort to equalize calories out to the new calories in.

The body is actually fighting against fat loss!

I'll let Guyenet explain:

> "Fat mass is biologically regulated. So, it's not just the result of conscious decisions to eat less or exercise more or eat more. It's a biologically regulated process. ... It has been shown in a number of studies in both animals and humans that if you restrict calories, you can produce fat loss. There's no doubt about that. You also produce a loss of lean body mass. **But as soon as you allow that animal or person to eat as much as they want to eat again, they bounce right back up to their original fat mass.** And that occurs whether you start with someone who is overweight or someone who is lean. **So, at least short-term changes in fat mass are compensated for very quickly by the body, and there are a number of mechanisms that are designed to pull fat mass back into the place where the body wants it."**[484]

Thus, the "burn more calories than you take in" approach to fat loss fails because it ignores the simple fact that your biology is *wired* to *prevent* you from actually succeeding in burning more calories than you take in for any significant length of time.

---

484 Kresser, C. (2010). Episode 1 – Stephan Guyenet on causes and treatment of obesity. Podcast retrieved from http://chriskresser.com/podcast-episode-i-interview-with-stephan-guyenet-on-obesity-and-weight-loss.

Here is the basic principle of how the body fat set point system operates:

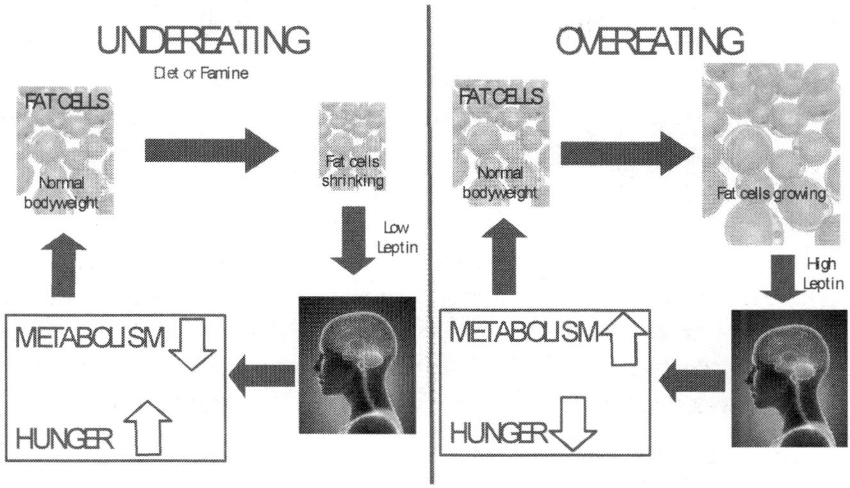

In essence, your fat cells are in constant feedback with your brain through a hormone secreted by the fat cells known as leptin. (More body fat = more leptin in the blood. Less body fat = less leptin in the blood.) As fat cells are depleted (during either a famine or, more likely in the modern world, a weight loss diet), the brain gets the signal that the body is being starved and then acts to survive the period of food shortage—by first increasing hunger, and then, if you don't eat, it decreases energy expenditure. During a period of overeating, the set-point system does the opposite in order to drive body fat levels back down. Overweight and obesity arise when this system becomes dysfunctional and begins defending higher and higher levels of fat mass.

Thus, rather than simply trying to forcibly starve the body of calories and engage in a fight against our own biology, we need a fundamentally different approach. As Guyenet explains,

"If there's one thing that's consistent in the medical literature, it's that telling people to eat fewer calories isn't a very effective fat loss strategy, despite the fact that it works if strictly adhered to. … Therefore, what we need for sustainable fat loss is not starvation; we need a treatment that lowers the fat mass set point. There are several criteria that this treatment will have to meet to qualify:

1) It must cause fat loss
2) It must not involve deliberate calorie restriction
3) It must maintain fat loss over a long period of time
4) It must not be harmful to overall health"[485]

What he has outlined here are the fundamental principles for long-term fat loss success—these four principles are the blueprint to a new scientific approach to lasting fat loss.

The seven nutrition strategies discussed in this chapter are all congruent with those four principles of resetting the body fat set point. It's not about simply starving the body of calories—it's about using dietary principles that lower fat mass *without* engaging in a fight against our own biology. But we also believe there are several non-diet (and non-exercise!) strategies that are critically important as well—such as NEAT (non-exercise activity thermogenesis) and circadian rhythm optimization. There are large bodies of research suggesting that chronically disrupted circadian rhythm/sleep deprivation and decreased NEAT are *major* factors in the obesity epidemic—perhaps just as important as changes in the food supply—and while we are addressing solely nutrition in this book, we believe it's important to make sure people do not approach fat loss as being solely a matter of diet, or diet and exercise, but to address all aspects of lifestyle that influence body fatness.

We would like to re-emphasize Guyenet's second principle listed above: **"It must *not* involve *deliberate* calorie restriction."**

Why might that be?

After all, in this book, we have made the case that calories, rather than the inherent metabolic effects of specific macronutrients, are the source of fat gain. So one might legitimately ask the question: **Why not just recommend counting calories and eating below a certain level of calories each day?**

Why do we recommend focusing on food quality over a simple and direct focus on calories?

Simple. While forced and deliberate calorie restriction can work for some people, it doesn't work for most.

---

485 Guyenet, S. (2010, January 31). The body fat setpoint, part iv: Changing the setpoint. Retrieved from http://wholehealthsource.blogspot.com/2010/01/body-fat-setpoint-part-iv-changing.html

We already know that when we put people either on weight loss diets that are at a fixed calorie level (telling them to count calories and never eat more than a given number of calories) or a diet where we tell people to eat however much food they want while sticking to certain food choices, the well-designed ad libitum diet dramatically outperforms that fixed calorie diet.

The reason for this is simple: the spontaneous reduction in calorie intake that occurs on ad libitum diets that focus on food choices is *different* than the reduction in calories that comes simply from relying on conscious effort and willpower to eat fewer calories. **The former works with your biology, and the latter works against it.** That is, fat loss from forced calorie restriction will engage all sorts of negative compensatory biological mechanisms (hunger pangs, fatigue, metabolism/NEAT decrease, etc.) that make it so you're fighting against your own biology as you're trying to lose fat. On the other hand, eating in a way that allows you to eat to fullness and not consciously/forcibly restrict calories does not seem to create these negative biological adaptations to anywhere close to the same degree. Instead of fighting against your fat loss efforts, the body actually seems to *want* to decrease fat mass and return to a leaner body fat set point in that environment.

The single biggest predictor of successful lasting weight loss is *hunger.*[486] Thus, what we need is not fat loss in the context of constant fighting against hunger pangs. What we need for lasting fat loss success is a strategy that causes fat loss *without hunger*. This is the difference between simple forced calorie restriction and strategies that drive ad libitum fat loss.

Eventually, we all end up eating ad libitum. Forced calorie restriction can only be sustained for so long before someone gives in to their body's desire to eat. It's miserable to fight hunger every day. So most of us eventually give in and give our body what it's demanding. Thus, the ideal is to adopt dietary and lifestyle principles that coax your body into a state of burning more calories than you consume *while minimizing/eliminating negative metabolic adaptations* (hunger pangs, decreased metabolic rate, decreased NEAT, fatigue, etc.). Well-

486 http://www.ncbi.nlm.nih.gov/pubmed/23512619?dopt=Abstract&holding=npg

designed ad libitum diets that adhere to the nutrition principles laid out in this chapter do that much more effectively than simple calorie restriction.

SUSTAINABLE DAILY DIETARY STRATEGIES ARE THE ROYAL ROAD TO SUCCESS

"You will never change your life until you change something you do daily."
- John C. Maxwell

The solution to fat loss is NOT any sort of short-term diet or exercise program. It is found in your daily habits!

For many of you, this is likely a major shift in your frame of reference *away* from the mentality of "How can I do __________ 30-day diet and exercise program to lose the fat?" to "How can I systematically incorporate better *permanent* habits into my life that will reliably lead to fat loss, without suffering?"

Sustainability is *not just* a simple matter of how difficult you consciously feel the strategy to be. This is a matter of biology. To the extent that you've adopted strategies for weight loss that lead to compensatory metabolic adaptations—decreased thyroid hormone, slowed metabolic rate, decreased NEAT, increased hunger, fatigue, etc.—these things will slowly alter the calories in, calories out equation in such a way that over time, despite your best efforts to continue restricting your diet and working out, fat loss will come to a screeching halt and you will slowly regain all the fat you lost.

To accomplish sustainable fat loss, you must:

1) **Choose strategies that are not psychologically arduous and do not rely on you constantly doing things that you find difficult and not enjoyable.**
2) **Adopt strategies that create fat loss while eliminating the negative metabolic adaptations that predispose you to future weight gain—that is, you want to work with your biology as much as possible, instead of engaging in a fight against it. The other factors mentioned in this section give you a good start on that—particularly with regard to nutritional factors.**

The essential strategy here is making sure that you have, first of all, put habits into place that ***do*** actually cause fat loss (such as lowering food reward and food variety, increasing protein intake, increasing plant and micronutrient intake, eating a mostly whole-food diet), and then make sure you are doing those things at a level that doesn't feel like suffering to you, and which you can sustain for the rest of your life without struggle.

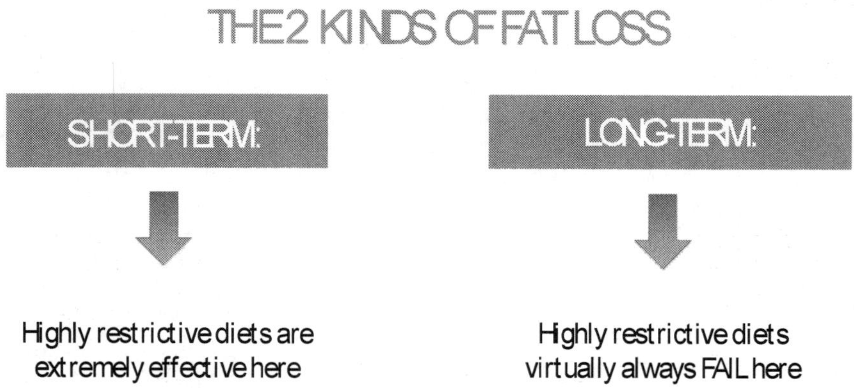
THE 2 KINDS OF FAT LOSS
SHORT-TERM:
LONG-TERM:
Highly restrictive diets are extremely effective here
Highly restrictive diets virtually always FAIL here

If your goal is only temporary fat loss, like for a physique competition or photo shoot, and you don't intend to maintain the fat loss, then a highly restrictive (unsustainably restrictive) diet is perfectly appropriate. But if you are one of the many millions of people who wants to lose fat and maintain it, or keep progressively losing more fat, then let me be very clear. **You should NOT be on a diet that consists of habits that are so difficult and unsustainable that you can only manage to do them for a few weeks or months at the most.** At best, you're wasting your time with such an approach (since you will inevitably regain the fat when you return to your normal habits), and at worst, the cycles of weight loss and regain will actually make you fatter over time. You want to shoot for a balance of doing enough of the habits known to produce fat loss in a way that can be sustained while being self-compassionate and flexible enough to allow for the inevitable indulgences that we all engage in occasionally. Compliance is the crux of lasting fat loss.

Having said that compliance is the key, we have created a useful model to help you understand the relationship between compliance on different types of diets and fat loss. On one end of the compliance spectrum, we see that the easiest diet to maintain is the Standard American Diet full of processed junk food. On the other end of the spectrum, the diets with the poorest compliance are the ones that ask for the most extreme deviation from that norm—very low-fat diets, vegan diets, diets that require avoidance of long lists of forbidden foods, and very low-carb (ketogenic) diets. The more extreme, the lower the compliance.

We conceptualize this as a spectrum of the Standard American Diet with perfect compliance on one end and any number of extremely restrictive diets with poor compliance on the other end.

STANDARD AMERICAN DIET
• Obese bodies
• Effortless compliance
EXTREME DIETS
(low-fat, vegan, very low calorie, very low carb)
• Lean bodies
• Terrible compliance

Right now, this is the predicament we find ourselves in. We can do what most people in our society do—which is the easiest thing to do and requires the least effort to maintain—and end up fat and sick as a result. Or we can choose to adopt one of the countless extreme fad diets with little chance of long-term success.

What you want is to implement the strategies to the point where you are actually achieving fat loss, but also simultaneously not feeling like you're suffering—you are not constantly battling hunger pangs, cravings, fatigue, etc.

Each person needs to find the optimal balance of establishing new habits that actually work for fat loss without experiencing carbophobia, fat-o-phobia, animal food phobia, starvation, suffering, deprivation, emotionally dysfunctional relationships with food, or constantly fighting hunger pangs.

Every person will fall into a different place on this spectrum in terms of what feels reasonable or possible to them, with some effortlessly creating new habits and others thinking that it is utterly "impossible" to break free from their current obesogenic behaviors. Ideally, the sweet spot is the point where you can comfortably add positive habits and reduce negative habits while not suffering. The goal is to find this sweet spot where your efforts are both effective and sustainable.

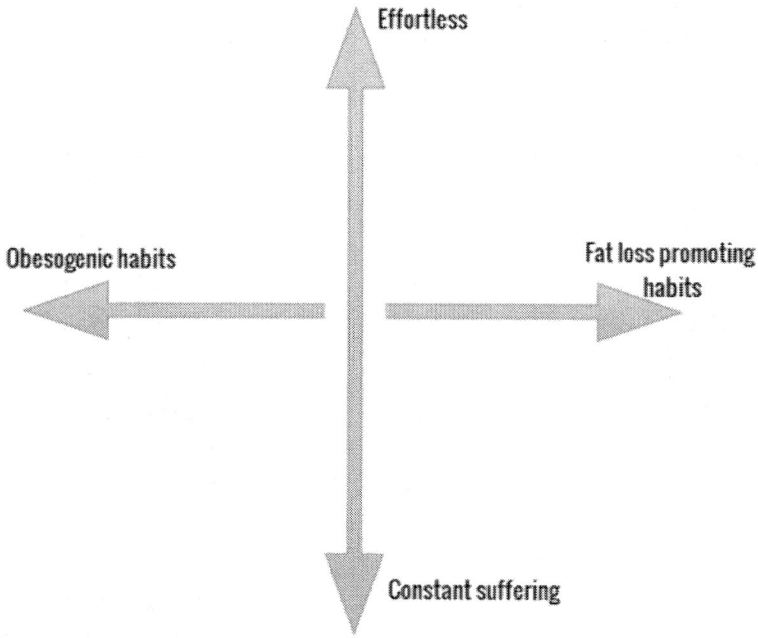

This shows you four different quadrants of where you can be in terms of your habits and how much ease (or suffering) you have in maintaining those habits.

To fill this in, it looks like this:

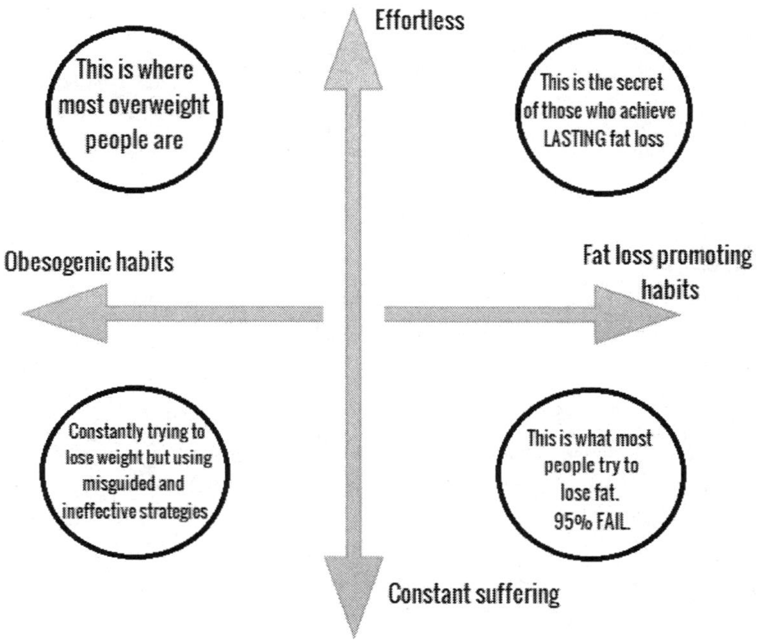

Upper left quadrant - Most overweight people are in a state of having obesogenic habits and are continuing those habits effortlessly.

Lower left quadrant - There are also some overweight people who are actively trying to lose weight, but who are using misguided or ineffective strategies and thus are needlessly suffering while not getting results. For example, there are some notable low-carb gurus who are still extremely overweight after years of extreme and highly restrictive low-carb diets. And when they fail to get results, instead of realizing that the approach is flawed, they often restrict carbohydrates even more. This is because they have fundamentally misunderstood that their body composition is a function of overall caloric balance, not the effects of carbohydrates or insulin.

Lower right quadrant - Most people who want to lose fat adopt completely unsustainable practices like low-calorie diets, juice fasts, crash diets, fad diets, crazy intense exercise regimens, extremely restrictive diets, low-fat diets, calorie counting, and other forms of intense restriction- and deprivation-based exercise and diet regimens. These require constant fighting against hunger pangs and cravings, overcoming fatigue, dealing with the effects of slowed metabolic rate, and, in general, constant willpower to continue to forcibly deprive yourself. This is why 95% of people fail to achieve lasting fat loss—they approach fat loss with a short-term, quick-fix mentality and adopt totally unsustainable practices. This is NOT where you want to be.

Upper right quadrant - Instead, you want to be in the upper right quadrant with a set of habits that promote fat loss (think the previous six factors I have mentioned in this section), and you want to be able to do those habits with as much effortlessness and ease as you do your current set of habits.

The bad news is that habit change isn't easy. It takes effort and willpower to establish any sort of new habits in your life—whether it's waking up earlier to start a meditation or exercise routine, or changing your diet. We are creatures of habit, and it is indeed hard work to establish any sort of new habit in basically any area of our lives. But the good news is that once you do put in this initial effort to perform that new habit for a period of time, then the new habit becomes automatic! Meaning, it actually takes *less* effort to continue that habit than to revert to the old habit. (Some automaticity research indicates that the average amount of time to establish a new habit is about 65 days,[487] but it varies individually, so it may take shorter or longer for you[488] to get to the point where the habit becomes automatic. It isn't easy for many people, but it absolutely can be done.)

This is the real secret of lasting weight loss. The magic isn't found in the perfect macronutrient ratio of carbs to fat or avoidance of one food group. It is found in following the above six factors—"eating wholesome foods in sensible combinations," as Katz would say—and implementing those as habits that you continue to do for the rest of your life.

If you want to achieve lasting fat loss, consider these words from obesity researcher Yoni Freedhoff, MD:

> **"My weight management philosophy has always been rather straightforward— whatever you choose to do to lose your weight, you need to keep doing to keep it off, and therefore choosing a weight loss modality you don't enjoy is just a**

---

487 http://www.resolutiontweet.com/focus-on-daily-habits-and-know-the-facts-about-21-days/

488 http://atlantaholisticmedicine.com/docs/How%20Habits%20are%20Formed.pdf

> **recipe for regain. ... [T]here is one essential commonality for those who succeed where others fail—if you're going to keep it off you've got to like how you've lost it enough to keep doing it."[489]**

SUMMARY

Overall, the research is very clear that the ratio of carbohydrates to fat in the diet simply doesn't matter all that much. The vast majority of studies show no differences in fat loss (or very minor, barely significant differences) between diets that vary dramatically in macronutrient content. In the long run, everything from Atkins high-fat, low-carb diets, to vegan high-carb, low-fat diets, to Mediterranean diets, and everything in between have about the same results in terms of improvement of body composition. The science simply does not support all the hype and claims over various low-carb diets or low-fat diets or the damaging health effects of one macronutrient or another. Contrary to the last several decades of myopic fixation on the amount of fat or carbohydrate in our diets, the research generally shows that carb and fat composition of your diet doesn't matter all that much.

What does matter is:

- **The effect of a dietary pattern on overall caloric balance** (i.e., if it actually causes fat loss).
- **Sustainability of that dietary pattern** (i.e., causes fat loss through means that one can sustain for life, while minimizing/eliminating negative metabolic adaptations).

In general, the most effective way to modify caloric balance of the diet is not through changing the quantity of various macronutrients in the diet. (Although all sorts of low-carb, vegan, and low-fat diets can work--to the extent that they inadvertently lower overall caloric intake.)

Nor is the best path to modifying caloric intake of the diet simply to count calories and forcibly restrict them below a certain level—since we know that, because of the way that different types of food affect us neurologically, there will be dramatic differences in hunger, lethargy, and satiety levels with different types of food even at the same caloric intake. (Naturally, dietary patterns that promote greater satiety, less

---

489 http://www.weightymatters.ca/2014/06/is-it-really-scientifically-impossible.html

hunger, and better energy levels at a given calorie intake will be most sustainable.)

Thus the best way to make sure your diet is promoting fat loss is not through a focus on either macronutrients (carbs versus fat) or through conscious calorie counting and restriction, but rather, the best way is through manipulating overall food quality—specifically factors like food reward, food variety, plant food intake, micronutrient density, and protein intake.

Chapter 10: It's Time to Move Beyond the Battle of the Macronutrients into the New Era of Health and Fat Loss

Pop quiz:

Carbs or fat—which of these can you eat as much as you want of without gaining fat?

a. Fat doesn't make you fat, carbs do!
b. Carbs don't make you fat, fat does!
c. You can eat both carbs or fat with impunity and neither can ever make you fat.
d. Both of these macronutrients can potentially make you gain fat if you are consistently overconsuming calories beyond your needs. There is no evil macronutrient, and no magical macronutrient that transcends the laws of thermodynamics.

If you answered "D," then give yourself a nice pat on the back. You are on the right path.

The wrong paths are represented by the common "hot" promises seen repeatedly on the internet and in most current diet books:

- "If you eat low-fat, you can eat whatever you want because fat makes you fat."
- "If you eat low-carb, you can eat whatever you want because carbs make you fat."

- "If you go on my juice cleanse, you will cleanse yourself of toxins, and then you will reset your metabolism and get to eat however you want because toxins make you fat."
- "If you cut out allergenic foods from your diet, you will get to eat whatever you want because allergens make you fat."
- "Cut out these five fattening foods, and you can eat however much you want because those foods put you in fat-storing mode."
- "Go on my carb cycling plan and you will get to 'cheat your way to being lean' and eat however you want."

Who doesn't want to get to exercise as much gluttony as they want and gorge themselves all the time without having to worry about fat gain? What better way to sell a book than to promise that it will only require a small amount of denial of one food group or another, and then you can indulge in all the gluttony you want and still lose weight and be healthy!

Unfortunately, it just isn't true.

Contrary to popular claims by nutrition gurus of various persuasions, there is an enormous body of scientific evidence that shows that when calories are kept equal, there are no differences in fat gain or fat loss in those who eat low-fat or low-carb.

There is no evil macronutrient whose consumption leads to fatness. Not fat and not carbs.

There is also no magical macronutrient that gives you the supernatural power of eating huge quantities of it without gaining fat. Neither a low-fat diet nor a low-carb diet grants you this ability.

Nope, carbs are not evil. Not starch. Not wheat. Not insulin. Not even sugar.

Nope, eating a low-carb, high-fat diet does not bestow any magical effects on you that allow you to circumvent evil "fat-storing" hormones or to transcend the laws of thermodynamics.

So what is really better for health and a lean body—low-carb or low-fat diets?

Neither!

The truth is that anyone who is operating from a framework of whether low-carb or low-fat is best is operating in the Stone Age of nutritional thought.

We have learned much about the science of proper nutrition over the last 30 years, and, simply put, we know that the answer to health and fat loss does not lie in the extent to which our diet is "low-fat" or "low-carb." These are overly simplistic concepts that don't have any place in the world of modern nutrition research.

It is well established in the science at this point that dietary fats run the gamut from good to bad to ugly, and that carbohydrates do too.

One cannot equate the omega-3 fats in seafood, or the monounsaturated fats in avocados, or the saturated fats in coconut oil, to, say, the omega-6 fats from soy oil or the trans fats in margarine. It is silly to lump these all under one semantic umbrella and try to lower intake of all those things called "fats."

Likewise, it is equally vapid thinking to lump everything from Snickers candy bars and doughnuts to carrots, yams, and blueberries under "carbs" and then try to "lower your carb intake."

The biggest factor that dictates how fattening the food you eat is is not the amount of carbs in your diet. Nor is it the amount of fats in your diet. Nor is it the carbohydrate versus fat ratio. Nor is it the amount of sugar or high-glycemic carbs in your diet. A focus on any of the above factors is a foolish diversion from the factors of real importance.

What are those factors that you *should* be focusing on?

Eating *real* food and consuming ample plant foods, and doing so with a focus on the seven strategies outlined in the previous chapter.

Once you're doing that, then you can concern yourself with macronutrient variation all you want without going wrong.

You can choose to eat a lower-carb diet that is rich in animal foods in addition to those plant foods, or a low-fat diet that is almost entirely plant foods. Both approaches are consistent with experiencing leanness and good health.

Dr. Katz has done one of the most extensive analyses of the scientific data on all the different popular diets out there, from low-carb, high-fat diets, to veganism, to low-fat omnivorous diets, to Mediterranean diets, to low-glycemic diets, to traditional Asian diets, to Paleo diets, and everything else you can think of—perhaps one of the most, if not *the* most, important nutrition study ever conducted to date. Based on all of this research, he concluded:

> **"The aggregation of evidence in support of (a) diets comprising preferentially minimally processed foods direct from nature and food made up of such ingredients, (b) diets comprising mostly plants, and (c) diets in which animal foods are themselves the products, directly or ultimately, of pure plant foods—the composition of animal flesh and milk is as much influenced by diet as we are—is noteworthy for its breadth, depth, diversity of methods, and consistency of findings. The case that we should, indeed, eat true food, mostly plants, is all but incontrovertible."** [490]

We already know that a high-fat diet full of processed junk foods and vegetable oils will generally lead to poor health and a fat body. We also already know that a high-carb diet full of processed junk foods and refined sugars will generally lead to the same poor health and a fat body. Contrary to what many low-carb gurus would have you believe, the science shows over and over again that there isn't anything magical about a low-carb diet.

- **You don't get any magical fat loss effect by removing oranges and carrots from your diet in favor of fatty meat, nuts, and oils.**
- **There is no mystical metabolism-boosting effect of eating a low-carb, high-fat diet. You don't lower your risk of obesity, diabetes, or heart disease by choosing butter and steak over blueberries and sweet potatoes.**
- **There is no extra fat loss that takes place on low-carb diets beyond what the calorie content of that diet dictates.**
- **There is no incredible energy boost that you get from burning fat instead of carbohydrate.**
- **Eating fat certainly does not transcend basic laws of thermodynamics and make you immune to getting fatter if you eat more calories than you're burning each day.**
- **There are no examples of Blue Zone populations around the world renowned for their incredible health and longevity who eat low-carb, high-fat diets. (There are**

---

490 http://www.annualreviews.org/doi/abs/10.1146/annurev-publhealth-032013-182351

numerous examples of such populations who eat high-carb, lower-fat diets.)

- **Carbs aren't the devil. And dietary fat is not a savior that bestows incredible health upon us while magically melting off our body fat.**

The simple fact is that if the claims from low-carb gurus about the effects of carbohydrates and fat were true, these things would be incredibly easy to identify with very basic controlled experiments. They would be extremely clear and obvious. If these claims about the damaging effects of carbs and the wonders of low-carb diets were true, countless studies would have validated them even 30 or 40 years ago when these things were first being tested. If well-controlled studies had shown that eating a low-carb, high-fat diet was *the* superior diet for general health, fat loss, performance, or longevity, we would have known about it—and it would've been well accepted by everyone in the scientific community—decades ago. All obesity scientists, physicians, and athletic coaches would accept that carbs and sugars—not calories—have been making us fat, diabetic, and worsening our performance all along. And they would all be telling us at every opportunity they had to get rid of any carbs in our diet—it would be standard practice for everyone to eat ultra-low-carb ketogenic diets. Sports coaches would have all their elite athletes eating ultra-low-carb ketogenic diets, and any athlete who wasn't eating this way would've been left in the dust long ago for not being able to keep up with the athletes running on the superior fuel of ketones. Obesity scientists, doctors, and dieticians would all be telling us to stop all this silliness of going to the gym to burn off calories, stop trying to eat fewer overall calories, avoid high-carb plant-based diets like the plague, and just focus on eating fewer of those evil carbs.

Yet, none of these things is the current reality.

Why?

Well, it's either because all the scientists conducting these studies for the last several decades are all incompetent and all the hundreds of experiments showing no difference between low-carb and high-carb diets (or differences in favor of higher-carb diets) are all wrong, or it's because the claims of low-carb advocates are wrong.

Which one makes more sense to you?

Overall, if there is any effect at all from manipulating one's carb to fat ratio, we are talking about an effect that is so utterly small that countless studies have failed to identify any significant difference at all—in terms of health, treating insulin resistance, athletic performance, and fat loss.

The truth is that the low-carb movement has lots of hype and devout followers but very little scientific substance. If there is anything we can conclusively say about diets that vary in their carb to fat ratio and how that relates to overall health and vitality, it's that the extremes of restricting either fat or carbohydrates (very low-fat diets and very low-carb diets) are likely to lead to worse results than a diet amply rich in all three macronutrients.

Overall, what the majority of research on the subject of low-carb, high-fat diets versus low-fat, high-carb diets indicates is not that either of these diets is radically superior to the other—it's that we've been looking for answers is the *wrong place!*

The answer to good health, optimal vitality, disease prevention, and high performance is not found in the extent to which our diet is low in carbs or high in carbs, or low in fat or high in fat. The actual value of manipulating your carb to fat ratio isn't anywhere even remotely close to what many low-carb gurus (and low-fat gurus, for that matter) would have you believe.

In our opinion, the whole anti-carb and anti-fat movements that have sought to blame our ills on one particular macronutrient should be piled on top of other crude and primitive medical relics like leeches and bloodletting. They are remnants of the Stone Age of nutritional thought. And rather than continuing to operate from this fundamentally flawed paradigm and search for the answer to our health and obesity woes through the extent to which our diet is low or high in carbs or fat, we ought to be laughing at ourselves that we ever approached nutrition in this way at all!

This whole carbs versus fat debate has been nothing but a useless distraction that has blinded us for decades from the real nutritional factors that dictate our health and body composition.

Thus, rather than continue the macronutrient wars, we suggest a shift in the modern conversation about nutrition, health, and fat loss. Let us move past carbs versus fat.

It is not carbs or fats that are ruining our health and making us fat. What is ruining our health and making us fat is poor food quality, highly rewarding processed food, low consumption of fruits and vegetables, lack of sleep and chronically disrupted circadian rhythm, lack of movement, and the desperate attempt to solve our health woes by extreme and unsustainable diets.

The focus on macronutrients above all else is fundamentally misguided.

The answer to better health and a leaner body is not to be found in any of the extreme diets out there with long lists of forbidden food groups and forbidden macronutrients.

As Katz puts it,

> **"I think it's time to stop talking about macronutrients, because people can cut carbs and eat badly, people can cut fat and eat badly, they can cut sugar and eat badly. Or you can cut carbs and eat well, or cut fat and eat well. ... The focus on macronutrients has been a decades-long boondoggle. The answer is wholesome foods in sensible combinations. You do that, and the macronutrients will take care of themselves."**[491]

This means a diet consisting of whole, unprocessed, nutrient-rich foods, with ample plant foods, and ample amounts of *all three* macronutrients gotten from whole foods. This can be done in hundreds of different ways that vary tremendously in macronutrient ratios, so what matters is that you follow the principles outlined in the previous chapter and find the way that feels good to ***your*** body and the way that allows ***you*** to sustain that way of eating and fully reap the rewards of nutrient-rich whole-food diets.

Don't become stressed and neurotic about the carb to fat ratio of your diet. The science simply doesn't warrant it. Focus on eating nutritious whole foods while following the 7 principles outlined in the previous chapter. Once you're doing that, you can feel free to move more towards the higher carb or lower carb end of the dietary spectrum without going wrong. Experiment with different types of whole foods (rich in all of the three macronutrients) and find a way of eating wholesome foods following the principles outlined in this book

491 http://live.smashthefat.com/do-calories-count-with-david-katz/

that you can turn into habits that are sustainable for the rest of your life.

Enjoy your food, enjoy your life, have enough energy to do what you want to do, and if all this nutrition talk makes you hungry, go eat something!

Eat fat! It's delicious and serves vital roles in your body.

Eat protein! It's delicious and serves vital roles in your body.

Eat carbohydrate! It's delicious and serves vital roles in your body.

It is no mistake that we are designed to find these substances tasty and that we crave these nutrients when they are lacking in the diet. Our bodies function best with an ample supply of all three macronutrients.

Oh, and if you've been low-carb for the last several years and you now find yourself with fatigue and various unexplained symptoms, eat something sweet. You'll feel better.

Free Test to Uncover the Hidden Factors Holding You Back From Losing Fat

In this book, we debunked the myths and pseudoscience around fat loss nutrition, and we showed you the real nutrition factors that determine your fat loss destiny. Now that you have a rock-solid understanding of the nutrition factors that determine your body fatness, it's still critically important to realize that fat loss is not *solely* determined by nutrition! As we cautioned earlier in the book, don't fall into nutrition myopia and get wrapped up in the never-ending pursuit of the *magic* diet that just melts the fat away. If you're already eating well, but you're still not losing fat, it's likely that you have other non-nutrition factors holding your fat loss efforts back.

Ari Whitten has developed a special test (which is 100% *free)* that is designed specifically for the purpose of identifying which factors are holding you back from losing fat. The test will tally up your answers and give you a personalized result showing you exactly what factors are holding you back. It also comes with a free ebook--*Unstuck: The 6 Potential Factors Sabotaging Your Fat Loss Efforts, and How to Fix Them*--that will explain more about the specific factors that the test identifies as problematic for you, and give you science-backed information on how to start fixing the problem. If you want to lose fat, this test will show you how to do it in the smartest and most efficient way possible.

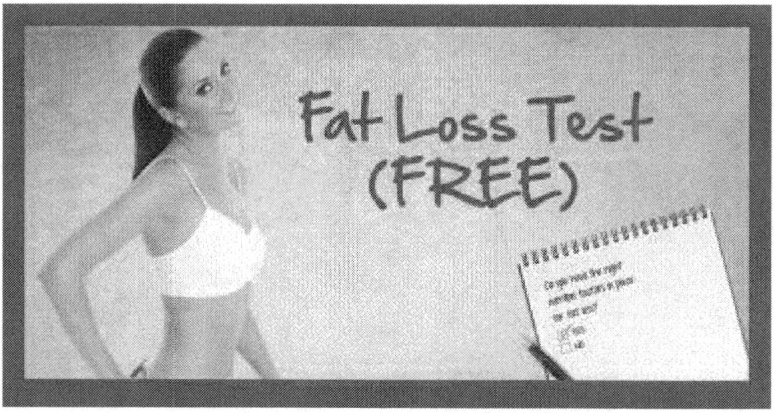

Go to the link below to take the TEST.

http://www.ariwhitten.com

Help Us Help Others

The information in this book can change the paradigm in the fat loss industry and can show people a real path to sustainable leanness. It can potentially help prevent millions of people from going on fad diets and spinning their wheels, torturing themselves while achieving nothing but worse health and an even slower metabolism. But in order to do that, this information has to reach more people, and that depends on you! So please do us a big favor and write a review for this book on Amazon. The more 5-star reviews it gets, the more this information will help others just like you escape from diet myths and pseudoscience and transform their lives. Thank you so much for reading our book. We sincerely hope you will use this information to transform your life. We also hope you will leave a review and help others do the same. We greatly appreciate the time and effort you put into writing thoughtful reviews!

About the Authors

Ari Whitten

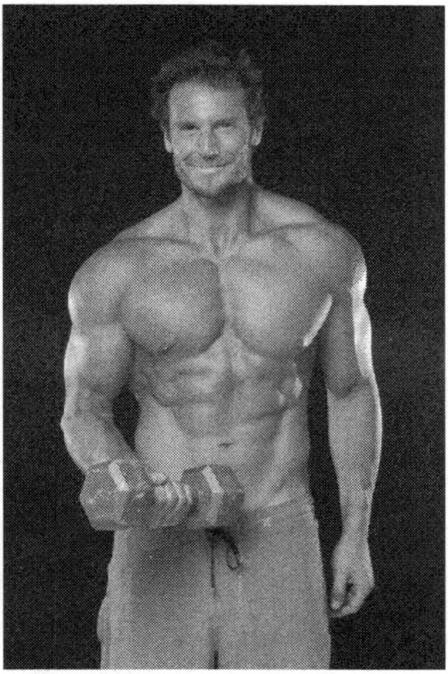

Ari Whitten is the #1 bestselling author of the cutting-edge book, *Forever Fat Loss*. He is a fat loss and nutrition expert who has been running a nutrition counseling and personal training business for over a decade. Ari has a Bachelor's of Science from San Diego State University in Kinesiology with a specialization in fitness, nutrition, and health. He holds two advanced certifications from the National Academy of Sports Medicine and recently completed coursework for his PhD in Clinical Psychology, an education which rounds out all aspects--nutrition, fitness, and psychology--of his approach to optimal health.

Ari is a tireless researcher who has obsessively devoted the last two decades of his life to the pursuit of being on the cutting-edge of the science on health, fitness, and nutrition. Ari's work is geared toward one purpose: To get effortless and permanent fat loss by working with your biology, rather than the painful and temporary fat loss one gets through programs that work against your biology. That is the focus of this book, as well as Ari's more advanced programs, such as *The Metabolism Supercharge* program (which is designed specifically for those with metabolic dysfunction and thyroid issues) and *The Forever Fat Loss Formula*. His other programs can be found on his website (www.ariwhitten.com).

The future of fat loss has arrived, and it's no longer about deprivation and willpower--it's about *biology*! Stop trying to fight against your biology and start working *with* your biology.

Dr. Wade Smith, MD, FACS

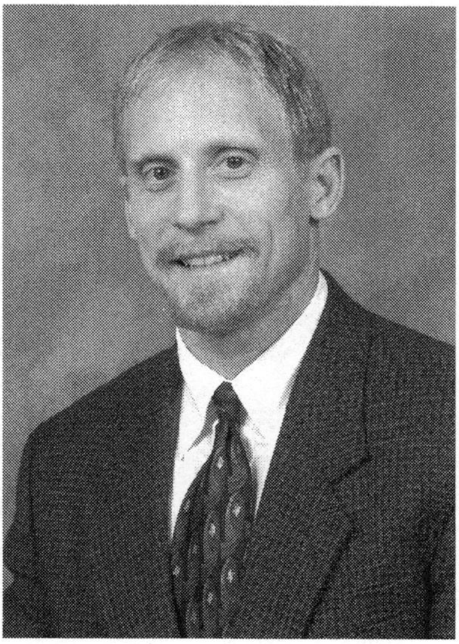

Wade Smith MD, is an Orthopedic Trauma Surgeon at the Swedish Medical Center in Englewood, Colorado and a Professor of Orthopedic Surgery at the University of Colorado, School of Medicine. He has an extensive background in the care and rehabilitation of injured patients, athletic injuries and athletic training and sports nutrition. He has competed at the International and national championship levels in Ice Hockey, Short Track Speedskating, Cycling and Bodybuilding. He has served as a physician in chief for USA Speedskating and cares for severely injured athletes as part of his daily clinical practice. Dr. Smith is active in research and regularly teaches at local, national and international levels. He has published over 150 peer reviewed scientific articles and written several textbooks. He serves on the editorial boards of numerous scientific and medical journals and is a senior member of the American College of Surgeons Committee on Trauma. His work in assisting injured patients to regain their life and health has led him into the fields of nutrition and health, with an emphasis on lifestyle changes to improve well-being and reduce susceptibility to disease. Dr. Smith is the editor in chief of Qangl, a patient advocacy healthcare website: www.qangl.com.

39997711R00200

Made in the USA
San Bernardino, CA
08 October 2016